SUPPORTING CHILDREN'S MENTAL HEALTH AND WELLBEING

This key text recognises the importance of upskilling students and practitioners to understand children's holistic needs and to develop new ways of working therapeutically that support their wellbeing and resilience.

The book outlines why therapeutic approaches are necessary, considers the range of approaches that are available and the evidence behind them and shows how these can be used to support children and families in an increasingly challenging practice landscape. Placing an emphasis on self-care, it celebrates the role of the practitioner as an inspirer of hope and architect of resilience and self-efficacy. Each chapter in the book:

- Provides an overview of adversity, trauma and holistic wellbeing
- Includes helpful case studies and practical examples, alongside reflective questions that can be used as discussion points in seminars
- Takes a multi-disciplinary approach with contributions from specialists working directly with children and families across a range of settings
- Equips students and practitioners with a wide range of models, tools and approaches to achieve their best outcomes
- Offers advice for developing a therapeutic relationship, and the skills and dispositions needed for practice.

This informative and practical book will be essential reading for students in a range of disciplines, including early years professional practice and early childhood degrees, as well as education, health, social care and community services. It will also be a valuable resource for early years and primary practitioners, trauma-informed schools and organisations supporting children and families.

Dr Alison Prowle is a senior lecturer at the University of Worcester, where she specialises in teaching and research connected to trauma-aware practice and children's adverse life experiences. Prior to joining the university, Alison worked extensively in schools, third-sector organisations and local authorities. Alison completed her doctoral studies at Cardiff University where her research focused on multi-agency and community support to forced migrant families in Wales. Alison has also undertaken extensive research with care experienced families, families with a disabled child and families in 'left behind' communities. She is passionate about equipping the children and family's workforce to use strength-based, democratic and compassionate approaches to support children and families to achieve positive outcomes and realise their aspirations.

Nicola Stobbs was a senior lecturer and course leader for the BA (Hons) Early Childhood in Society at the University of Worcester. The degree was underpinned by Social Pedagogy, a human-rights based approach focusing on ethics, relationship-based practice and empowerment. She has undertaken considerable research with groups experiencing adversity and marginalisation, for example kinship children and carers, children and families in areas of deprivation and Roma, Gypsy Travellers. Before working at the university, Nicola was a primary school teacher and the manager of a pre-school. Nicola is also the chair of Play Worcester, a charity committed to ensuring children have opportunities to play outside more often in their communities.

SUPPORTING CHILDREN'S MENTAL HEALTH AND WELLBEING

Therapeutic Approaches for Working with Children and Families

Alison Prowle and Nicola Stobbs

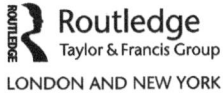
Taylor & Francis Group
LONDON AND NEW YORK

Designed cover image: © Getty Images

First published 2025
by Routledge
4 Park Square, Milton Park, Abingdon, Oxon OX14 4RN

and by Routledge
605 Third Avenue, New York, NY 10158

Routledge is an imprint of the Taylor & Francis Group, an informa business

© 2025 Alison Prowle and Nicola Stobbs

The right of Alison Prowle and Nicola Stobbs to be identified as authors of this work has been asserted in accordance with sections 77 and 78 of the Copyright, Designs and Patents Act 1988.

All rights reserved. No part of this book may be reprinted or reproduced or utilised in any form or by any electronic, mechanical, or other means, now known or hereafter invented, including photocopying and recording, or in any information storage or retrieval system, without permission in writing from the publishers.

Trademark notice: Product or corporate names may be trademarks or registered trademarks, and are used only for identification and explanation without intent to infringe.

British Library Cataloguing-in-Publication Data
A catalogue record for this book is available from the British Library

ISBN: 978-1-032-60569-2 (hbk)
ISBN: 978-1-032-60568-5 (pbk)
ISBN: 978-1-003-45966-8 (ebk)

DOI: 10.4324/9781003459668

Typeset in Interstate
by codeMantra

CONTENTS

About the authors   vii
List of figures   viii
List of tables   ix
Preface   x

PART I
Understanding the needs of children and families   **1**

1   An introduction to working therapeutically with children and families   3

2   Understanding adversity   17

3   Supporting the holistic needs of children and families   32

PART II
Exploring therapeutic approaches to supporting children and families   **47**

4   The importance of play   49

5   The role of creativity in supporting those who have experienced adversity   62

6   The great outdoors   77

7   A mindful approach   90

8   Talking therapies   102

9   The power of stories   119

PART III
Enhancing the role of the practitioner in supporting children and families   **131**

10   The attuned practitioner   133

| 11 | Supporting our own wellbeing | 147 |
| 12 | Bringing it all together and next steps | 161 |

| *Index* | 167 |

ABOUT THE AUTHORS

Dr Alison Prowle is a senior lecturer at the University of Worcester, where she specialises in teaching and research connected to trauma aware practice and children's adverse life experiences. Prior to joining the university, Alison worked extensively in schools, third-sector organisations and local authorities. Alison completed her doctoral studies at Cardiff University where her research focused on multi- agency and community support for forced migrant families in Wales. Alison has also undertaken extensive research with care-experienced families, families with a disabled child and families in "left behind" communities. She is passionate about equipping the children and family's workforce to use strength-based, democratic and compassionate approaches to support children and families to achieve positive outcomes and realise their aspirations.

Nicola Stobbs was a senior lecturer and course leader for the BA (Hons) Early Childhood in Society at the University of Worcester. The degree was underpinned by Social Pedagogy, a human-rights based approach focusing on ethics, relationship-based practice and empowerment. She has undertaken considerable research with groups experiencing adversity and marginalisation, for example kinship children and carers, children, and families in areas of deprivation and Roma, Gypsy Travellers. Before working at the university, Nicola was a primary school teacher and the manager of a pre-school. Nicola is also the chair of Play Worcester, a charity committed to ensuring children have opportunities to play outside more often in their communities.

FIGURES

2.1	Life adversities	17
2.2	Stress response	24
3.1	The three psychological needs	42
4.1	Simplified version of the Learning Zone Model (from Stobbs, 2019)	50
5.1	Four characteristics of creativity	63
8.1	CBT triangle	105

TABLES

1.1	Potential effects of factors contributing to poor mental health on two parental life trajectories	7
3.1	Potential risk factors of insecure attachments between child and parent/caregiver	33
3.2	Head, Heart and Hands, what's missing?	41
3.3	Head, Heart or Hands; what does each situation call for?	41
4.1	Levels of tolerance of risk using the three Ps	51
5.1	A conceptual model of the four stages of psychosocial transition from trauma incorporated into art therapy, based on Appleton's Avenues of Hope (2001)	68
5.2	Evidence of aspects of creativity found in the case study and the benefits of them	73
6.1	Reflection on the benefits of the outdoors	85
7.1	Reflection on a mindfulness activity	96
10.1	Perspectives on taking a therapeutic approach to a child experiencing a disorganised attachment	142
11.1	Boundaries, strategies and rationale for improved wellbeing	156
12.1	Personal action plan based on learning from each chapter	166

PREFACE

This book was born out of a deep commitment to helping practitioners, students and trainees from a range of different backgrounds, contexts and disciplines to understand the complex challenges faced by many children and families, and to respond with empathy and effectiveness. When we were designing a new course, with a therapeutic approaches module, we searched high and low for a textbook that combined strong underpinning theory with practical approaches. We couldn't find exactly what we were looking for, and so we decided to write this book!

The book is presented in three parts. Part I, Understanding the needs of children and families, sets the scene with three theoretical chapters which highlight the issues that children and families face, the contexts in which they live and the importance of positive mental health and wellbeing. Part II, Exploring therapeutic approaches to supporting children and families, consists of a series of chapters which each focus on a different therapeutic approach. Within this section you will discover a range of evidence-based approaches, from play to CBT strategies, each designed to meet the diverse needs of children and families. Case studies and practice vignettes throughout the book provide additional insight from a range of practitioners. Readers are invited to engage in reflective tasks and to challenge themselves with critical questions. Part III, Enhancing the role of the practitioner in supporting children and families, concludes the book, with a focus on practitioner wellbeing, self-care and professional development. Throughout the book, we draw on social-pedagogy principles, strength-based approaches and trauma-informed practice consonant with our value base.

We hope that this book serves as a resource and an inspiration, equipping you with the tools and approaches needed to help make a positive difference to the children and families you work with.

Alison and Nicola

Part I
Understanding the needs of children and families

1
An introduction to working therapeutically with children and families

Introduction

The evidence is indisputable; in the UK children's mental health is declining while the number of child referrals to mental health support services are rising. Referrals for very urgent mental health support were 43 percent higher in June 2024 than June 2023 (Barron & Williamson, 2024). Clearly community and health services are falling behind in real terms, resulting in missed opportunities for early intervention and stressful waits for children and families with the potential deterioration of health and wellbeing, all of which affect children and young people's everyday quality of life and their long-term life chances (Community Network Survey, 2023). So, how did we get to this point, and what can be done?

Social, political and cultural factors

There is no one reason why the nation's wellbeing is so low and mental health problems are increasing, but the evidence suggests that there has been a perfect storm of national policy intersecting with local contexts with impacts on individuals. Below we explore some theories.

Social media

Although there is a small correlation between social media use and mental health issues (Orben, 2020) the issue is not clear cut because much depends on how social media is used. Evidence suggests that whether the user is active or passive makes a difference. Some have found that those who actively like, share and comment on posts tend to find social media a positive influence, contributing to their social capital and reducing isolation (Verduyn et al., 2017), while those who are passive may experience envy and negative social comparisons (Burke et al., 2010). Another study contested this perspective, however, suggesting that social media was beneficial to wellbeing only when participants used it as a tool to talk to family and friends (Burke & Kraut, 2016). It may be that the effects of engaging with social media varies across time and context and the same users who find it beneficial on some occasions may also find it harmful to mental health on others (Burke & Kraut, 2016).

Educational stress

In 2003, West and Sweeting controversially proposed that schools were having harmful effects on children's mental health. Over 20 years later, the Good Childhood Report found that school was still a worry for children (The Children's Society, 2024).

Bourdieu proposed that schools classify children by testing and sorting them for future positions (Bradbury & Swailes, 2022). This is particularly pertinent in modern, knowledge societies where educational attainment is used to filter applications for jobs. Lack of academic success, therefore, impacts on personal identity, self-worth and self-esteem (Landstedt et al., 2009) as well as children's everyday experience of school because their future prospects, both economic and social, are dependent on their performance in high stake tests and exams (Banks & Smyth, 2015). With more children hoping to study for a degree, and with much knowledge building on previous understanding, pressure to perform well affects children from a young age (Putwain, 2009). These stresses can result in anxious transitions from adolescence to adulthood and insecurity about life trajectories (Pinquart et al., 2014).

COVID-19

From March 2020 until March 2021 the UK was under lockdown restrictions as part of efforts to control the spread of COVID-19. For people already prone to anxiety the additional worry of contracting the disease, potentially fatally affecting not only themselves but also others through inadvertently passing it on, was intensified, resulting in fear, confusion, social isolation and anger (Brooks et al., 2020). Due to the closure of businesses, many became unemployed and fell into debt, known causes of depression (Paykel, 2003).

There were some children and families, however, who reported higher wellbeing during lockdown as they enjoyed more family time, maintained regular sleep patterns (no late-night socialising), worried less about bullying and had more control over when tasks were done (Soneson, 2023).

The extent to which the COVID-19 pandemic affected mental health was largely determined by the circumstances people were in before it began. Those most at risk were those with pre-existing mental health conditions, coping with adverse childhood experiences (ACEs) (see Chapter 2 for more on this), being a victim of racism or discrimination and loneliness (Mental Health Foundation, 2020).

Austerity

Following the worldwide financial crash in 2008 and the resulting economic recession the UK government pursued policies of austerity in an attempt to control public sector debt to avoid a financial crisis. This meant reduced spending on public services such as health, education and prisons, and increases in tax.

The connection between austerity and wellbeing is widely known. As discussed, unemployment and debt can lead to depression (Paykel, 2003); mental health issues are exacerbated when poor housing and social deprivation are added to the mental health mix, frequently resulting in individuals self-medicating with alcohol and drugs, leading to despair, further isolation from society and poor physical health (Knapp, 2012). These results should be interpreted cautiously, however, as people with mental health issues are also more likely to be unemployed, leading to financial worries and social isolation, and therefore anxiety and depression (Knapp, 2012), so it is difficult to unpick any causality.

Income inequality

The income gap between rich and poor has widened steadily over the past 30 years. Perhaps unsurprisingly researchers have found a "a compelling quantitative association between income inequality and depression" with the impact felt nationally, locally and individually (Patel et al., 2018, p.86).

National inequality

As governments adopt austerity measures, failing to invest in public housing, health, education, transport, pollution control and the availability of nutritious food, those who are dependent on these services, with no ability to avail themselves of alternatives, are at a heightened risk of depression (Patel et al., 2018 p.85). The situation worsens over time, for example, if rental properties are not monitored and damp is not tackled, tenants are at risk of serious physical health problems, as well as associated mental health issues. Inequality therefore perpetuates more inequality as less spending on health leads to more despair and depression.

Local level

As some social groups become very much wealthier than others, those in poorer groups can feel inferior and defeated in comparison (Buttrick & Oishi, 2017). When some people manage to improve their circumstances, but others do not, this inequality is experienced as deep frustration and anger and can sometimes culminate in local protests and riots, contributing to anxiety and depression (Burns et al., 2017).

Income inequality also erodes local social capital by threatening social cohesion within communities. As higher educated people leave poorer neighbourhoods there is a reduction in the availability of cognitive skills, knowledge and information that can be utilised to communicate with and influence those in power, which contributes to feeling forgotten (Vilhjalmsdottir et al., 2016). These communities are sometimes referred to as "left behind communities". Others prefer the phrase "held back communities" (All Party Parliamentary Group (APPG), n.d.) because they are held back by government policies and experience the effects of inequal distribution of economic, social and technological opportunities (APPG, n.d.). Income inequality therefore affects perceptions of fairness (Buttrick & Oishi, 2017). Children and young people are particularly affected by income inequality in communities because this is the time of life when social trust and identity is developed. It is also the age when mental health problems begin to emerge (Patel et al., 2018).

Individual level

Individuals living in communities of high deprivation contend with scarce local services and facilities such as parks, pubs, libraries, shops, community centres and transport infrastructure that other areas often take for granted (APPG, n.d.). This is experienced individually as psychological stress, social defeat and depression (Pickett & Wilkinson, 2015), particularly in societies like ours that promote meritocracy (the idea that anyone can succeed by their own abilities) and the expectation that life will be better for us than it was for our grandparents (Roex et al., 2019). Culturally, the difficulties these individuals experience are blamed on them.

Increased awareness

Foulkes and Andrews (2023) propose that increased awareness of mental health issues has conversely contributed to its rise through both *improved recognition* and *overinterpretation*.

Mental health awareness raising campaigns aim to encourage more people to seek help and treatment and have prevented further illness and death by suicide (Henderson et al., 2017). There are, however, side-effects of increased awareness and the resultant change in societal attitudes. Campaigns may inadvertently contribute to the 'psychiatrisation' of what Freud called ordinary human unhappiness (Brinkmann, 2014, p.2). Campaigns may imply that disclosing episodes of depression or struggles with anxiety is a courageous and worthy thing to do (Kosyluk et al., 2021). This potentially endows social value to suffering from mental health challenges, which may be attractive to some people (Foulkes & Andrews, 2023).

Because of improved recognition many people are self-diagnosing their mental health conditions using social media, the internet and newspapers as sources (Lane, 2020); small symptoms are dwelt on and magnified until they become serious (Tekin, 2011). The individual's self-identity and behaviour changes as a result and professionals treat the 'new' person as having a mental disorder, resulting in a self-fulfilling prophecy (Hacking, 1996).

As access to professional physicians becomes more difficult and waiting lists grow longer self-diagnosis is likely to become more prevalent. While this will be an accurate diagnosis and increase self-knowledge and treatment options in some cases, in others it may worsen what might have been a temporary wellbeing blip through overinterpretation of symptoms (Lane, 2020). This is particularly relevant for educating children in school about mental health and wellbeing as studies have shown that some efforts to promote mindfulness or cognitive behavioural therapy (CBT) have negatively impacted on pupils' wellbeing, when it was not low to begin with (Andrews et al., 2023; Garmy et al., 2015).

Ironically, as the number of people diagnosed with mental health conditions increases (self or clinician diagnosed) more campaigns raising the awareness of mental health conditions are launched. As we have discussed, however, these efforts increase rates of mental health issues, thus one compounds the other and the cycle perpetuates (Foulkes & Andrews, 2023).

Mental health and young children – the need for action

We often assume that childhood is a carefree time and that the mental health challenges arise in adulthood. Sadly, a significant minority of children experience poor mental health in their early years. In 2019, for example, 100,000 children (5.5 per cent) aged 2-4 years in England struggled with anxiety, behavioural disorders and neurodevelopmental disorders. Globally, a staggering 20.1 per cent of children aged between 1 and 7 have a mental health condition including anxiety disorder (8.5 per cent), depressive disorder (1.1 per cent), oppositional defiant disorder (4.9 per cent) and attention-deficit hyperactivity disorder (ADHD) (4.3 per cent), with 6.4 per cent experiencing more than one mental health condition (Vasileva et al., 2021).

Risk factors are prevalent before a child is born; smoking, alcohol or substance abuse during pregnancy all contribute to the development of a mental health condition for the baby, and once the baby is born factors such as domestic violence and abuse compound the issue (Royal College of Psychiatrists, 2023). This is significant because mental health issues in early childhood are an indicator of future mental health challenges (Liu et al. 2017; Ziegler et al., 2023).

Given the long-term implications of adversity in childhood, we can see why doing nothing is not an option.

Ghosts in the nursery

We must guard against judging families with mental health issues harshly and remember that parents generally try to do their absolute best for children, but parents' previous history can impact on their capacity to offer children a good start in life. Fraiberg et al. (1980) refer to this as "ghosts in the nursery … visitors from the unremembered past of the parents" (p.164). Fraiberg found that if parents were shown empathy rather than condemnation and supported to process their childhood experiences therapeutically, "the ghosts depart, and the afflicted parents become the protectors of their children against the repetition of their own conflicted past" (p.196).

REFLECTIVE TASK

Consider the likely life trajectory of two children born in different circumstances. Complete Table 1.1 by writing what the effects each factor may have on mental health problems. The first one has been done for you as an example.

Table 1.1 Potential effects of factors contributing to poor mental health on two parental life trajectories

Contributing factor	Child born to a self-medicating mother in deprived circumstances	Child born to a mother in more affluent circumstances and with a good social network
Social media	Mother sees images of 'perfect' families; it adds to her depression and sense of hopelessness.	Mother enjoys engaging with her NCT group online and sharing tips. She feels connected and able to cope.
Educational stress		
COVID-19		
Austerity measures		
Income inequality		
Increased awareness of mental health factors		

Critical questions

1. Which factor had the biggest impact on mental health?
2. Were any factors interrelated?
3. How much difference did you attribute to the circumstances of a child's birth?
4. If you answered, 'it depends on …' for each situation, what does this tell us about how we should work with children and families?

The need for practitioners to be upskilled in therapeutic approaches

During early childhood the brain is at its most to malleable, offering the best opportunity for successful intervention to prevent children developing mental health issues, enable them to have fulfilling adult lives and contribute to society (Royal College of Psychiatrists, 2023). This means that those working with children and families can influence outcomes for children that go beyond educational attainment. Using non-specialist practitioners to deliver community-based interventions, such as providing resilience building activities (see Chapter 4 for more on resilience) or supporting parents to bond with their children, has been identified as a way of preventing many mental health problems developing into full-blown clinical conditions (Patel et al., 2016). Taking a therapeutic approach to your practice is a key part of this prevention process.

What is a therapeutic approach?

The word 'therapeutic' is related to the treatment of diseases and healing (*Cambridge Dictionary*, 2025). Taking a therapeutic approach when working with children and families, therefore, means looking behind the behaviour presented, considering why the child may be displaying that behaviour and then drawing on various approaches to enable them to heal from the cause of their dysregulation.

As professionals we are key mediators between unloving home environments, with the associated negative impact on children's behaviour, and society's expectation of conformity to social norms (Charles, 2019). We act as a bridge whereby "the child can find himself reflected in the eyes of someone who sees him as an individual and also expects him to meet certain standards of community behaviour" (Charles, 2019, p.158). Adopting a therapeutic approach does not mean permitting unacceptable behaviour but appreciates that when there is unresolved trauma and grief the development of a stable self-identity has been hindered. Adopting an informed, therapeutic approach can interrupt the cycle of trauma (Charles, 2019, p.157).

 Case study: Ruth Bullock – therapeutic foster parenting

The following case study is by Ruth Bullock, a trained therapeutic foster carer who forms part of a therapy team. She is committed to providing a loving and accepting home for trauma-experienced children who cannot live with their birth parents. Here she discusses her experience of therapeutic parenting.

> There is often a misconception that being therapeutic means not imposing discipline or boundaries. Children who spent their early years in environments where adults didn't make them feel safe actually crave consistent boundaries but enforcing them must be trauma informed. A child who associates raised voices with violence will not learn healthy responses if a harsh style of parenting is adopted.
>
> The main challenge of a therapeutic approach is that it takes time. This can be frustrating and there are times when it feels like it isn't working because you can't see the benefits overnight. When a child is in crisis and constantly dysregulating, it can often feel impossible to respond therapeutically.
>
> Asserting authority with a child experiencing trauma before a safe bond has been established is triggering to the brain and children respond as they would have done in previous unsafe situations, fight, flight, freeze, fawn or flop. A child who has experienced trauma will use all these responses depending on the threat so we, as the safe adult, must know the child on a deep level to recognise the signs of each response.
>
> I learned strategies from the fostering therapeutic team and was amazed at the impact one of the simplest strategies had. After explaining to a team member that I had used every strategy I knew with a little boy who was often physically dysregulated, particularly towards me, I was asked "Have you tried asking him if he just needs a cuddle?" At the time it seemed like a ridiculous question to ask. Had she not listened to the extreme behaviours I was facing? What I didn't realise was that this was the first step for him to learn that he could ask for physical reassurance and it would be given. This hadn't happened to him before. The physical touch, the regulation of my breathing against his, the tight feeling of my arms wrapped around him, helped his physical response return to calm and de-escalated the trigger. All he needed was to feel safe.

Critical questions

1. Based on Ruth's experiences how would you explain what a therapeutic approach is?
2. What is difficult about this approach?
3. What are some key components for success?

Three approaches to therapeutic work

There are generally three main therapeutic approaches that professionals ascribe to and although you do not need to formally adopt a particular stance it can be helpful to be informed about each of them.

Psychodynamic approach

This school of thought considers a person's early experiences to be critical in the development of identity and personality. One of its key founders, Freud, advocated listening very attentively, both to what is said and what is not said and therefore being potentially repressed. This makes clinical observation skills critically important because behaviour cues, emotional states and the non-verbal interactions of babies and young children are indications of what they cannot express in words (Royal College of Psychiatrists, 2023). In practice this means being skilled in listening to children about their anxieties through their silence, or how they speak through their disruptive behaviour (Charles, 2019).

There is much that will resonate with practitioners, but the approach is not without critique. Some point out that it is impossible to verify what a non-talking child thinks, while others suggest there is an implication that individuals are slaves to their pasts and have no influence on changing their life course (MacBlain, 2018).

Person-centred approach

Carl Rogers is the founder of a person-centred approach and is most well known for the phrase 'unconditional positive regard'. Two other associated concepts are 'congruence', meaning that we should be completely genuine in our relationship with others, and 'empathy' where we try to feel as the other person feels. In this approach there is no attempt to interpret a person's thoughts for them or direct them in to a 'right answer', rather the therapist helps them work out what might be preventing them from leading a fulfilling life and then unblock it (Cooper & McLeod, 2011).

Some, however, have questioned whether we can categorically say that all humans are worth "unconditional positive regard", for example, individuals who commit atrocities. Others point out that the unstructured nature of the approach may not be suitable for everyone, while others have suggested that practitioners may be masking acceptance and genuineness when this does not reflect their true feelings, for example, when working with abusers (Masson, 1992).

Cognitive approach

Cognitive behavioural therapy (CBT) (see Chapter 8 for more on this) is based on the premiss that our thoughts and behaviour are interrelated. If our actions are determined by our thoughts and vice versa, changing our thoughts can change our behaviour (Pattison & Harris, 2006).

In practice this could involve using dolls, puppets or role play to explore various ways of responding to a situation. Restructuring negative thoughts into more positive ones is another option, for example, if a mother blames herself for her child's fussy eating, she might reframe this as remembering that she is raising someone who will become an adult and as long as she has taught them to feed themselves, they will make decisions about the food they consume. This prevents the individual from overly fixating on a negative view of themselves.

Exposure to the trigger might also feature in CBT, for example, if a child is anxious about dogs after a bad experience small exposures may be introduced such as stroking a toy dog, holding the lead of a dog and, finally, touching a real dog.

CBT has its critics too, with some arguing that it is mechanistic and focuses on issues in isolation (Gaudiano, 2008) and because of the emphasis on confronting emotions and thoughts it might not be appropriate for individuals with learning difficulties (NHS England, 2022).

Taking an integrative approach

There is merit in all the therapeutic approaches discussed and blending aspects of each as appropriate to each situation is arguably the best tactic (Aziz *et al.*, 2020). Taking a psychodynamic approach reminds us of the impact our early years has on long-term development and the crucial importance of cultivating observational skills. The person-centred perspective helps us bear in mind the significance of building genuine relationships with those we aim to help and drawing on elements of CBT can potentially help children and families feel empowered to change their own behaviour.

> ### Critical questions
>
> 1. Do you favour any of the approaches? If so, which ones?
> 2. Can recognise elements of these approaches in your practice?
> 3. If adopting an integrative approach, which parts would you take from each approach?

Implications of doing the wrong things

Although working therapeutically can guide our practice, we should retain an element of caution, particularly regarding safeguarding.

Taking a therapeutic approach may heighten the possibility that you will be exposed to safeguarding concerns, either through a child making a disclosure, or signs of abuse or other harm, for example, radicalisation. It is important not to jump to conclusions, but understanding your setting's safeguarding policy is critical and you must follow it to protect you, the child and the setting. The NSPCC's webpage is a useful resource if you need unbiased advice.

You should also be cautious about becoming overly optimistic and go beyond your remit as a non-specialist therapeutic practitioner. We cannot fix every difficult situation, and some individuals may have serious unresolved trauma and adversity where they need specialist intervention because their neurobiology has changed (Aguirre, 2023).

We must also refrain from saying things that we cannot be sure about, for example, "You will feel better in the morning", or "I'm sure your dad will visit this weekend". Making promises you cannot keep erodes trust and might make children less likely to keep their promises in the future (Kanngiesser *et al.*, 2017). This is illustrated in the practice vignette below.

 Practice vignette

Hannah is a professional working with trauma-experienced children. She is trained to remain calm and consistent, leaving space for feelings and restorative conversations after incidents of dysregulation, followed by a reiteration of boundaries and expectations. When working with two particularly challenging young children, Noah and Charlie, Hannah was confident that her professional skills would enable her to cope with their misbehaviour whilst remaining in control, so confident that she promised to never shout at them.

Hannah spent weeks building a loving relationship with Noah and Charlie and was consistently reliable and steady in her responses, apart from once when, in a moment of weakness, she raised her voice. Looking very pleased with himself Charlie declared, "See, I knew you would shout at me."

Hannah was heartbroken at this slip-up and realised that she had failed the test the boys had set to ascertain if she was utterly reliable. She never made a promise that she might not be able to keep again.

Critical question

What mistake did Hannah make in her work with Noah and Charlie?

Conclusion

In this chapter we have discussed the rising incidences of mental health issues and potential reasons for this. We highlighted how this was concerning because children are negatively impacted by their parents' poor mental health, being more likely to develop mental health concerns themselves in later years.

Potential causes were considered and the role that non-specialist therapeutic practitioners can play by appropriately applying therapeutic methods. This does not mean that they allow children to misbehave, but where there is a shortfall in children's capacity to regulate their behaviour, they maintain consistent regard for the child as a person of worth. In doing so practitioners may draw on all the main approaches of therapeutic work; psychodynamic, person-centred and cognitive but should be aware of professional boundaries and seek external support as appropriate. Safeguarding policy and procedures should always be followed, and practitioners should guard against making promises that cannot be met.

Although mental health issues in children are increasing at a worrying rate, with the right care and support many of these can be prevented (Royal College of Psychiatrists, 2023).

Introduction to therapeutic approaches: key points

- Child referrals to mental health support services are rising.
- There is no definitive reason why people are experiencing low wellbeing and mental health issues but there is evidence that social media, educational stress, COVID-19, austerity, income inequality and increased awareness are contributory factors.
- Poor mental health in parents impacts on their children's mental health.

- Parents' previous history can impact on their capacity to provide the best start in life for their children.
- Due to the long-term implications of this, failing to act is not an option.
- There is a growing need for practitioners to be upskilled in therapeutic approaches.
- There are three main approaches to therapeutic work; psychodynamic, person-centred and cognitive. An integrative approach is often beneficial.
- Using non-specialist therapeutic practitioners to deliver community-based interventions such as resilience building has been identified as a way of preventing many mental health problems developing into full-blown clinical conditions (Patel et al., 2016).
- Taking a therapeutic approach does not mean permitting unacceptable behaviour but understands that where there is unresolved trauma and grief therapeutic approaches should be adopted to help interrupt the cycle of trauma.
- Practitioners should not over-reach their remit and be aware of the implications of doing the wrong things. Safeguarding policy and procedures should always be followed.

ADDITIONAL RESOURCES

- Cooper, A. and McNulty, P. (2024) *Empty plates and cold homes: What it's like to grow up in poverty in 2024.* Available at: https://www.barnardos.org.uk/sites/default/files/2024-09/Barnardos%202024%20-%20Empty%20Plates%20and%20Cold%20Homes.pdf (Accessed 24 October 2024).

This Barnardo's report highlights the link between a family's poverty and their mental health.

- Frayman, D., Krekel, C., Layard, R., MacLennan, S. and Parkes, I. (2024) *Value for money. How to improve wellbeing and reduce misery.* London School of Economics and Political Science, and Centre for Economic Performance. Available at: https://cep.lse.ac.uk/pubs/download/special/cepsp44.pdf (Accessed 24 October 2024).

This report questions whether a government's success should be measured by the extent to which it increases its citizen's wellbeing. It examines initiatives such as putting mental health support into schools would offer value for money that would benefit both the economy and society.

References

Aguirre, L. (2023) Why CBT might not be working for you. Understanding trauma and the limitations of cognitive behavioral therapy. *Psychology Today,* Available at: https://www.psychologytoday.com/gb/blog/true-self-empowerment/202301/why-cbt-might-not-be-working-for-you (Accessed 16 January 2025).

All Party Parliamentary Group (APPG) (n.d.) 'Left behind' neighbourhoods: definition, experience, and opportunity. Available at: https://www.appg-leftbehindneighbourhoods.org.uk/report/left-behind-neighbourhoods-definition-experience-and-opportunity/#:~:text=The%20concept%20of%20'left%20behind,of%20a%20more%20globalised%20economy (Accessed 18 October 2024).

Andrews, J.L., Birrell, L., Chapman, C., Teesson, M., Newton, N., Allsop, S., McBride, N., Hides, L., Andrews, G., Olsen, N., Mewton, L. and Slade, T. (2023) Evaluating the effectiveness of a universal eHealth school-based prevention programme for depression and anxiety, and the moderating role of friendship network characteristics. *Psychological Medicine* 53(11), pp. 5042–5051. doi: 10.1017/S0033291722002033.

Aziz, M.O., Mehrinejad, S.A., Hashemian, K. and Paivastegar, M. (2020) Integrative therapy (short-term psychodynamic psychotherapy & cognitive-behavioral therapy) and cognitive-behavioral therapy in the treatment of generalized anxiety disorder: a randomized controlled trial. *Complementary Therapies in Clinical Practice* 39, May, 101122. doi: https://doi.org/10.1016/j.ctcp.2020.101122.

Banks, J. and Smyth, E. (2015) 'Your whole life depends on it': academic stress and highstakes testing in Ireland. *Journal of Youth Studies*, 18(5), pp. 598–616. doi: https://doi.org/10.1080/ 13676261.2014.992317.

Barron, J. and Williamson, S. (2024) Autumn Budget 2024: what you need to know. NHS confederation. Available at: https://www.nhsconfed.org/publications/autumn-budget-2024-what-you-need-know#:~:text=Additional%20funding%20for%20mental%20health,2024%20than%20in%20June%202023. Accessed 16 January 2025

Bradbury, A. and Swailes, R. (2022) *Early childhood theories today*. London: Learning Matters/Sage.

Brinkmann, S. (2014) Languages of suffering, *Theory & Psychology*, 24(5), pp. 630–648. doi: https://doi.org/10.1177/0959354314531523

Brooks, S.K., Webster, R.K., Smith, L.E., Woodland, L., Wessely, S., Greenberg, N. and Rubin, G.J. (2020) The psychological impact of quarantine and how to reduce it: rapid review of the evidence, *The Lancet*, 395(10227), pp. 912–920. doi: https://doi.org/10.1016/S0140-6736(20)30460-8.

Burke, M., and Kraut, R.E. (2016) The relationship between Facebook use and wellbeing depends on communication type and tie strength. *Journal of Computer-Mediated Communication*, 21(4), pp. 265–281. doi: https://doi.org/10.1111/ jcc4.12162

Burke, M., Marlow, C. and Lento, T. (2010) Social network activity and social wellbeing. *Proceedings on the SIGCHI Conference on Human Factors in Computer Systems*, 10–15 April, pp. 1909–1912. doi: https://doi.org/10.1145/1753326.1753613

Burns, J.K., Tomita, A. and Lund, C. (2017) Income inequality widens the existing income-related disparity in depression risk in post-apartheid South Africa: evidence from a nationally representative panel study. *Health Place*, 45, pp. 10–16. doi: 10.1016/j.healthplace.2017.02.005.

Buttrick, N.R. and Oishi, S. (2017) The psychological consequences of income inequality. *Social and Personality Psychology Compass*, 11(3), pp. 1–12. doi:10.1111/spc3.12304.

Cambridge Dictionary (2025) available online at: 16 January 2025).

Charles, M. (2019) Trauma and identity, in Charles, M. and Bellinson, J. (eds.) *The importance of play in early childhood education*, London: Routledge, pp. 150–159.

Cooper, M. and McLeod, J. (2011) Person-centered therapy: a pluralistic perspective. *Person-Centered and Experiential Psychotherapies*, 10(3), pp. 210–223. doi: https://doi.org/10.1080/14779757.2011.599517.

Foulkes, L. and Andrews, J.L. (2023) Are mental health awareness efforts contributing to the rise in reported mental health problems? A call to test the prevalence inflation hypothesis. *New Ideas in Psychology* 69, (101010), pp.1–6. doi:https://doi.org/10.1016/j.newideapsych.2023.101010

Fraiberg, S. (ed.) *Clinical studies in infant mental health: the first year of life*, New York: Basic Books, Inc., pp. 387–421.

Fraiberg, S., Adelson, E. and Shapiro, V. (1980) Ghosts in the nursery: a psychoanalytic approach to the problems of impaired infant-mother relationships, in

Garmy, P., Berg, A. and Clausson, E.K. (2015) A qualitative study exploring adolescents' experiences with a school-based mental health program. *BMC Public Health*, 15(1), pp.1–9. doi:10.1186/s12889-015-2368-z.

Gaudiano, B.A. (2008) Cognitive-behavioural therapies: achievements and challenges. *Evidence-Based Mental Health*,11(1), pp. 5–7. doi: 10.1136/ebmh.11.1.5.

Hacking, I. (1996) The looping effects of human kinds, in Sperber, D., Premack, D. and Premack, A.J. (eds.) *Causal Cognition: A Multidisciplinary Debate, Symposia of the Fyssen Foundation.* Oxford: Oxford University Press. doi: https://doi.org/10.1093/acprof:oso/9780198524021.003.0012.

Henderson, C., Robinson, E., Evans-Lacko, S. and Thornicroft, G. (2017) Relationships between anti-stigma programme awareness, disclosure comfort and intended help-seeking regarding a mental health problem, *British Journal of Psychiatry*, 211(5), pp. 316–322. doi:10.1192/bjp.bp.116.195867.

Kanngiesser, P., Köymen, B. and Tomasello, M. (2017) Young children mostly keep, and expect others to keep, their promises. *Journal of Experimental Child Psychology*, 159(July), pp. 140–158. doi: https://doi.org/10.1016/j.jecp.2017.02.004.

Knapp, M. (2012) Mental health in an age of austerity. *BMJ Mental Health*, 15(3), pp. 54–55. Available at: https://mentalhealth.bmj.com/content/ebmental/15/3/54.full.pdf (Accessed 14 October 2024).

Kosyluk, K., Marshall, J., Conner, K., Macias, D.R., Macias, S., Beekman, B. M. and Her, J. (2021) Challenging the stigma of mental illness through creative storytelling: a randomized controlled trial of this is my brave, *Community Mental Health Journal*, 57(1), pp.144–152. doi: 10.1007/s10597-020-00625-4.

Landstedt, E., Asplund, K. and Gillander Gådin, K. (2009) Understanding adolescent mental health: the influence of social processes, doing gender and gendered power relations. *Sociology of Health and Illness*, 31(7), pp. 962–978. doi: https://doi.org/10.1111/j.1467-9566.2009.01170.x.

Lane, R. (2020) Expanding boundaries in psychiatry: uncertainty in the context of diagnosis-seeking and negotiation. *Sociology of Health & Illness*, 42(S1), pp. 69–83. doi: 10.1111/1467-9566.13044.

Liu, X., Lin, X., Xu, S., Olson, S.L., Li, Y. and Du, H. (2017) Depressive symptoms among children with ODD: contributions of parent and child risk factors in a Chinese sample, *Journal of Child and Family Studies*, 26(11), pp. 3145–3155. doi: https://doi.org/10.1007/s10826-017-0823-4

MacBlain, S. (2018) *Learning theories for early years practice*. London: Sage.

Masson, J. (1992) *Against therapy*. London: Flamingo Publishing.

Mental Health Foundation (2020) *Coronavirus. The divergence of mental health experiences during the pandemic*. Available at: https://www.mentalhealth.org.uk/sites/default/files/2023-01/MHF%20The%20COVID-19%20Pandemic%202.pdf (Accessed 17 October 2024).

NHS Confederation (2023) *Waiting times in children and young people's services: Community Network survey*. Available at: https://nhsproviders.org/media/695836/cyp_survey_briefing-may-2023.pdf (Accessed 22 April 2024).

NHS England (2022) *Overview – cognitive behavioural therapy (CBT)*. Available at: https://www.nhs.uk/mental-health/talking-therapies-medicine-treatments/talking-therapies-and-counselling/cognitive-behavioural-therapy-cbt/overview/#:~:text=Some%20critics%20also%20argue%20that,such%20as%20an%20unhappy%20childhood (Accessed 23 October 2024).

Orben, A. (2020) Teenagers, screens and social media: a narrative review of reviews and key studies, *Social Psychiatry and Psychiatric Epidemiology*, 55(4), pp. 407–414. doi:https://doi.org/10.1007/s00127-019-01825-4.

Patel, V., Burns J.K., Dhingra, M., Tarver, Brandon, A.K. and Lund, C. (2018) Income inequality and depression: a systematic review and meta-analysis of the association and a scoping review of mechanisms, *World Psychiatry*, 17(1), pp. 76–89, doi: https://doi.org/10.1002/wps.20492.

Patel, V., Chisholm, D., Dua, T. et al. (eds.) (2016) *Mental, neurological, and substance use disorders: disease control priorities*. 3rd edn. Washington: World Bank Publications. doi:10.1596/978-1-4648-0426-7.

Pattison, S. and Harris, B. (2006) Counselling children and young people: a review of the evidence for its effectiveness. *Counselling and Psychotherapy Research*, 6(4), pp. 233–237. doi:10.1080/14733140601022659.

Paykel, E.S. (2003) Life events and affective disorders, *Acta Psychiatrica Scandinavica*, 108(s418), pp. 61–66. doi: 10.1034/j.1600-0447.108.s418.13.

Pickett, K.E. and Wilkinson, R.G. (2015) Income inequality and health: a causal review, *Social Science & Medicine* 128(December), pp. 316–326. doi: 10.1016/j.socscimed.2014.12.031.

Pinquart, M., Silbereisen, R.K. and Grümer, S. (2014) Perceived demands of social change and depressive symptoms in adolescents from different educational tracks, *Youth & Society*, 46(3), pp. 338–359. doi: https://doi.org/10.1177/0044118x11435575.

Putwain, D.W. (2009) Assessment and examination stress in key stage 4. *British Educational Research Journal*, 35(3), pp. 391–411. doi: https://doi.org/10.1080/01411920802044404.

Roex, K.L., Huijts, T. and Sieben, I. (2019) Attitudes towards income inequality: 'Winners' versus 'losers' of the perceived meritocracy. *Acta Sociologica*, 62(1), pp. 47–63. doi: https://doi.org/10.1177/0001699317748340.

Royal College of Psychiatrists (2023) *College Report CR238 – infant and early childhood mental health: the case for action*. Available at: https://www.rcpsych.ac.uk/news-and-features/latest-news/detail/2023/10/21/rcpsych-urges-government-to-act-as--children-under-five-face-lifelong-mental-health-conditions (Accessed 21 October 2024).

Soneson, E., Puntis, S., Chapman, N. et al. (2023) Happier during lockdown: a descriptive analysis of self-reported wellbeing in 17,000 UK school students during Covid-19 lockdown. *European Child and Adolescent Psychiatry*, 32(6), pp. 1131–1146. doi: https://doi.org/10.1007/s00787-021-01934-z.

Tekin, Ş. (2011) Self-concept through the diagnostic looking glass: narratives and mental disorder. *Philosophical Psychology*, 24(3), pp. 357–380. doi: 10.1080/09515089.2011.559622.

The Children's Society (2024) *The Good Childhood Report 2024*. Available at: https://www.childrenssociety.org.uk/sites/default/files/2024-08/Good%20Childhood%20Report-Main-Report.pdf (Accessed 16 October 2024).

Vasileva, M., Graf, R.K., Reinelt, T., Petermann, U. and Petermann, F. (2021) Research review: a meta-analysis of the international prevalence and comorbidity of mental disorders in children between 1 and 7 years, *Journal of Child Psychology and Psychiatry*, 62(4), pp. 372–381. doi: https://doi.org/10.1111/jcpp.13261.

Verduyn, P., Ybarra, O., Résibois, M., Jonides, J. and Kross, E. (2017) Do social network sites enhance or undermine subjective wellbeing? A critical review, *Social Issues and Policy Review*, 11(1), pp. 274–302. doi: https://doi.org/10.1111/sipr.12033.

Vilhjalmsdottir, A., Gardarsdottir, R.B., Bernburg, J.G. et al. (2016) Neighborhood income inequality, social capital and emotional distress among adolescents: a population-based study. *Journal of Adolescence*, 51(1), pp. 92–102. doi: 10.1016/j.adolescence.2016.06.004.

West, P. and Sweeting, H. (2003) Fifteen, female and stressed: changing patterns of psychological distress over time, *Journal of Child Psychology and Psychiatry*, 44(3), pp. 399–411. doi: https://doi.org/10.1111/1469-7610.00130.

Ziegler, M., Wollwerth de Chuquisengo, R., Mall. V. and Licata-Dandel, M. (2023) Early childhood mental disorders: excessive crying, sleep and feeding disorders, and interventions using the "Munich model" as an example, *Bundesgesundheitsblatt Gesundheitsforschung Gesundheitsschutz*, 66(7), pp. 752–760. doi: 10.1007/s00103-023-03717-0.

2
Understanding adversity

Introduction

Everyone experiences adversity at different points in their lives. Adversity can come in many forms such as personal loss, health challenges, financial difficulties or social conflicts. While the nature and severity of these experiences can vary greatly, facing and overcoming adversity is a common part of the human experience. How we respond to adversity can significantly shape our personal development and our outlook on life. Facing many adversities can be debilitating for the individual, and contribute to negative outcomes. However, it is often through the challenges of adversity that individuals develop resilience, learn valuable life lessons and grow stronger. In this chapter, we explore the diverse types of adverse experiences, their effects on children's lives and propose strategies that can mitigate their impact.

Adverse life experiences

The Merriam Webster Dictionary (2002) defines adversity as "a state or instance of serious or continued difficulty or misfortune". Everyone experiences adversity to some extent over the course of their lives. Figure 2.1 shows some common adversities that people face.

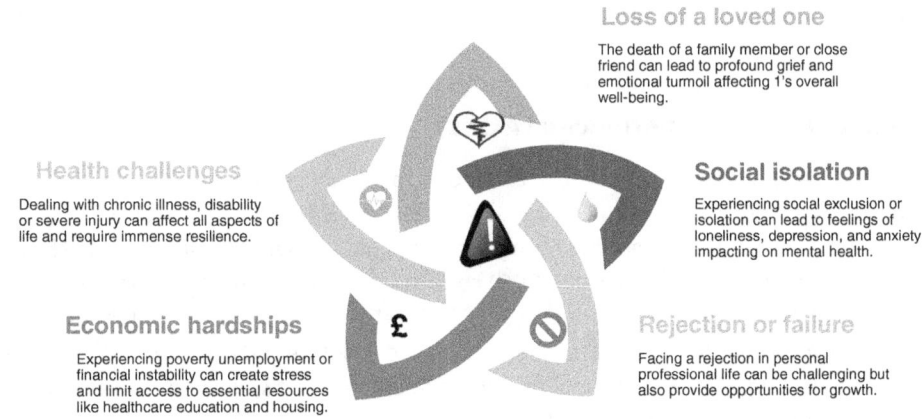

Figure 2.1 Life adversities

DOI: 10.4324/9781003459668-3

Helen Keller was an American author and disability rights advocate. She lost her sight and hearing at the age of 19 months, following a childhood illness. Despite the many challenges she faced, Helen learned to communicate, with the help of her teacher who taught her to read, speak and write. Speaking of adversity Helen Keller once said, "Although the world is full of suffering, it is also full of the overcoming of it" (Keller, 1903). In other words, whilst adversity is inevitable, we often find the capacity to overcome the challenges and achieve good outcomes. Throughout this book, we will be considering in more detail how children and families can be supported when facing life's challenges. The following strategies may help individuals manage and overcome difficult circumstances:

- Having an effective support network
- Regularly practising self-care
- Understanding and expressing feelings
- Setting small, achievable goals
- Focusing on what you can control
- Securing professional help when struggling.

Multiple adversities

Although adversity is a universal human experience, some individuals face multiple interconnected hardships that can be overwhelming and make it difficult to cope. Rankin and Regan (2004) describe such adversity as complex and interlocking challenges that individuals face, often spanning both health and social issues. This can include a combination of mental health problems, substance misuse, disabilities and social exclusion. Poverty can be a compounding factor within these adversities, with lack of resources making everything else more difficult to address. Rankin and Regan emphasise the breadth and depth of adversity. In other words, how many adversities are there, and how profound is their impact? Prowle and Musgrave (2018) also suggest that the longevity of adversity (how long the adversity lasts) can also have an impact on the extent to which people are able to cope with it, and move on to successful outcomes. Understanding the concept of multiple adversities emphasises the need for responsive, individually tailored and holistic approaches to support individuals dealing with these overlapping adversities. An example of multiple adversities is found in the case study later in this chapter.

Adverse childhood experiences (ACEs)

Child abuse, neglect and other adverse childhood experiences have long been associated with poorer health outcomes in adulthood (Springs & Friedrich, 1992). However, until recently, there was little research focused on the impact of multiple adversities. In a landmark study based in the United States, Felitti *et al.* (1998) considered the relationship between childhood experiences of adversity and negative health and wellbeing outcomes in adulthood. They defined ACEs as potentially traumatic events that occur before the age of 18 and may have profound and lasting effects on an individual's development and wellbeing. The researchers identified several ACEs ranging from physical, emotional or sexual abuse to neglect, household dysfunction and exposure to violence. They found that such experiences are common within the population, and have strong, cumulative effects on adult health, risk behaviours and diseases. The more ACEs an individual reported, they argued, the greater the risk of poor outcomes. The researchers also posited that the impact of ACEs can extend far beyond childhood, influencing mental and physical health, educational outcomes and social relationships well into adulthood. They suggested that understanding the nature and consequences of these adverse experiences is crucial for developing effective interventions and support systems to help children overcome challenges and build resilience. Versions of the ACEs study have subsequently been carried out in many other countries, including the United Kingdom (Bellis et al., 2014; Bellis et al., 2015: Bellis et al., 2019). The UK studies demonstrated that in parts of the United Kingdom around half of all adults identified that they had experienced at least one ACE, as defined by the original study (Felitti et al., 1998). By the age of 49, almost a quarter of those with high levels of ACEs (four or more) had been diagnosed with at least one chronic or life-limiting illness, whereas this was the case for only 6.9 per cent of those without ACEs (Bellis et al., 2015).

Whatever the causality, the correlation between childhood adversity and poor health in adulthood is evident. As such, the concept of ACEs has become very influential in policy and interventions to support children and families. The ACEs studies have been helpful in articulating a link between childhood adversity and its profound, long-term impacts. The studies have also been successful in making the case that financially investing in prevention and intervention in childhood adversity could have long-term benefits. The concept of ACEs also provides an easy to apply framework for practitioners to use in assessment and intervention.

However, it is worth noting that several criticisms have been levelled against ACEs theory (Hartas, 2019). The first challenge relates to the methodological design of ACE studies, which rely upon self-reported, retrospective data, which, by its very nature is highly subjective and prone to recall bias (remembering things inaccurately). The studies have also been criticised because most participants were white and middle class, and hence, the ACEs rarely focus on non-Western experiences of war, persecution, forced migration or starvation, and so fail to reflect the lived realities of many individuals.

Toxic stress and the 'toxic trio'

Whilst some stress can be helpful in motivating us or protecting us from danger, it is possible for the normal stress response to become damaged. Toxic stress refers to the prolonged activation of the stress response system. In the absence of positive and protective relationships, stress can disrupt the development of brain architecture and other organ systems, increasing the risk of stress-related diseases and cognitive impairments (Centre on the Developing Child, 2024). Environments that exacerbate stress include those with elevated levels of instability, violence and economic hardship. Left unchallenged, this combination of adversities can lead to significant developmental challenges and long-term health consequences for children.

The term 'toxic trio' is sometimes used to describe the stress that occurs when a particular combination of adversities affects a child's life concurrently. These factors are domestic abuse, substance misuse and parental mental health issues. These factors are often present in cases of child abuse and neglect, creating a highly adverse environment for children (Hood et al., 2021). A number of studies have suggested that where the toxic trio are present, the effects on children's wellbeing are particularly profound and long lasting, requiring significant intervention to help children overcome the odds whilst "changing the odds" (Hart et al., 2016, p.3).

Whilst the concept of the toxic trio can be helpful in identifying children who may be at risk of significant harm, the terminology can be very stigmatising for families. This theory has also been criticised because although studies often highlight the interrelationship of these three factors, they do not a explain how these factors interact or, indeed, how they can be helpfully addressed. The term toxic trio can oversimplify complex family dynamics. It may also lead to the assumption that the presence of these factors automatically results in abuse or neglect, which is not always the case. It should, therefore, be remembered that each factor is multi-faceted and can manifest in diverse ways in different families (Skinner et al., 2021). It is also noted (Prowle & Musgrave, 2018) that these adversities often coexist with further compounding factors such as poverty and social isolation. Focusing solely on the toxic trio can mean that other crucial factors that contribute to child welfare such as poverty, disability, culture or language barriers may be overlooked. Although there is evidence that the toxic trio can affect children adversely, responsive support services can help to mitigate these risks; a poor outcome is not inevitable if the right support is put in place. These criticisms of the toxic trio theory highlight the need for a more nuanced approach to understanding and addressing the factors that contribute to children's outcomes.

 Case study: Antoinette Frearson – understanding adversity (Part 1)

Antoinette Frearson is currently a doctoral researcher. She previously worked in a special school supporting young children's wellbeing and education. Antoinette says of this role, "It was extremely fulfilling and enjoyable. It was great to see the children grow, both developmentally and in their confidence, to live their fullest and most independent lives possible." This case study is presented in two parts. Part 1 of the case study, in this chapter, provides a rich example of Layla, a child facing adversity. (For the purpose of ensuring an ethical approach, all identifying details have been changed and Layla's story has been constructed from Antoinette's experience of supporting children over many years).

> Layla was only 18 months old when she and her baby sister were adopted. Before that, she lived in a flat with her mum who was addicted to drugs and alcohol. After Layla was born, doctors discovered that she was suffering from foetal alcohol poisoning. Sadly, as a young baby, in need of love, care and attention, she was left alone and hungry for extended periods of time. Social workers were aware of the situation, and Layla's mum was given many opportunities to get treatment for her addictions. Support was offered, such as a bed, cot and other essential household furniture, as well as money to buy food and baby formula. Unfortunately, she sold it all so she could buy more drugs and alcohol. It was heartbreaking reading Layla's notes, and imagining what she must have gone through, and how this shaped her perception of the world and her caregiver. I could also imagine how much her mum must have been struggling. What had happened to her in her past that had left her unable to cope with day-to-day life, dependent on alcohol and drugs to the point that she struggled to look after herself and her baby daughter? Layla was

being neglected, and she was starving. When the mum became pregnant for a second time, and as soon as Layla's baby sister was born, both children were adopted.

The girls' adoptive parents were a financially secure couple with lots of love to give. The girls now enjoyed food availability, shelter, love, care, and access to health services if feeling poorly – their needs were finally being met. Maslow (1954) clearly illustrated how important it is for these needs to be met in his Hierarchy of Needs model, and showed that without the basic needs of human life, which are so integral and fundamental to our existence, not only are we unable to survive, but we cannot thrive or move on to a place where we are fulfilling our potential and living our best life possible (self-actualisation). Each of these steps provide a good foundation and springboard to the next level, so if some needs are not being met, our foundations will be shaky, and we will not be able to become the best we can be. For the first time, the two girls had solid foundations and their physiological needs, safety needs and their need for love and belonging were being met. They were also being fully supported to thrive at school, make friends and start to plan for the future.

Layla's younger sister was doing just that. Despite having some additional needs (she had also suffered foetal alcohol poisoning), she was flourishing and achieving age-related expectations and had become well adjusted to her new life. She had formed a secure and early attachment to her adoptive mum. She made friends and had the capacity to enjoy holidays (temporary changes to routine) and independence as she grew and matured.

Layla also made some developmental improvements, but she had been older than her sister when she was adopted and had been more aware, on a visceral level, of being hungry and left alone with no-one responding to her cries for help. Consequently, she struggled to settle as well into her new home and situation and achieve developmental milestones. The school she was attending struggled to cope with her increasing needs, so she was given an Education, Health, and Care Plan (EHCP) based on a diagnosis of disorganised attachment disorder, and secured a special school place. Despite these struggles she was able to enjoy hobbies such as horse-riding and swimming, which she loved.

Critical questions

- From the description above, what do you see as Layla's needs and strengths? How might you seek to support those needs, and build on the strengths?
- As a practitioner, what skills, knowledge and understanding would you need to support Layla effectively? How long do you think it might it be before you see any improvement?
- Antoinette draws upon Maslow's Hierarchy of Needs model, when thinking about how best to support Layla. How helpful is this model in helping us understand children's needs? Are there any limitations to this model?

Part 2 of this case study is found in Chapter 10, where we consider the effectiveness of Antoinette's approach to supporting Layla.

Applying a strength-based approach

Whilst it is always important to identify risks, focusing on the strengths and resilience of families is crucial (Saleeby, 1996). Hodgkins and Prowle (2023) focus on identifying and levering the strengths of individuals, even in the most challenging situations. The approach aims to be optimistic and empowering for families, fostering resilience and positive outcomes by recognising and building on the family's own existing capabilities and resources. Their work emphasises the importance of seeing the glass half full and encourages practitioners to look for strengths rather than deficits, with the philosophy applied across various stages of development from early childhood to young adulthood.

Similarly, the Ecological Systems Theory proposed by Bronfenbrenner (1979) presents the child at the centre of nested systems which affect the child's wellbeing. Bronfenbrenner highlights the importance of considering multiple layers of influence when assessing and addressing child adversity. The theory examines how the different systems such as the family, school, community or wider social policy, interact with and influence a child's development. As Prowle and Musgrave (2018) point out the Systems Theory (Friedman & Allen, 2023) allows for a holistic consideration of the factors affecting children's wellbeing, including the ability to highlight strengths and needs within the system and target interventions effectively.

Understanding trauma

Distressing life events are often described as traumatic. However, within psychological trauma theory, it is not the event itself that represents trauma, but rather the individual's response to that event. This response is highly individual, and can be affected by previous life experiences, environmental influences and individual factors. This explains why two people may witness or experience the same upsetting event, but their trauma response is quite different. Psychological trauma then is an emotional response to a deeply distressing or disturbing event that overwhelms an individual's ability to cope. It can result from a single incident such as an accident or assault or from prolonged exposure to harmful situations like ongoing abuse and neglect. Some individuals experience complex trauma, which refers to exposure to multiple, often interrelated, traumatic events typically of an oppressive or interpersonal nature over an extended period. Complex trauma can deeply affect an individual's sense of self, emotional regulation and ability to manage relationships (Complex Trauma.org, n.d.). Trauma often leads to feelings of intense fear and helplessness and can have a significant impact on a person's mental, emotional and physical wellbeing.

Post Traumatic Stress Disorder (PTSD) in children is a mental health condition that can develop after a child experiences or witnesses a distressing event. Such events might include physical or emotional abuse, natural disasters, accidents or the loss of loved ones. Symptoms in children can differ from those in adults, and may include nightmares, flashbacks, severe anxiety or changes in behaviour such as becoming more withdrawn or conversely becoming more oppositional. It is important to recognise such signs and seek professional support to help the child cope and recover effectively. Early intervention is crucial, as it can significantly improve children's ability to cope and recover. Ongoing support from family, teachers and mental health professionals plays a vital role in helping children to navigate and heal from their trauma.

In a population level study in England and Wales, Lewis *et al.* (2019) found that 31.1 per cent of young people experienced trauma, and 7.8 per cent had developed PTSD by the age of 18. They reported that trauma-exposed young people were twice as likely to develop a mental health disorder as the general population. There was also a high prevalence among the trauma-exposed young people of self-harm and suicide ideation, often presenting alongside high-risk behaviours such as substance misuse. As Wadsworth (2015) highlights, such behaviours should be seen as (unaddressed) maladaptive coping mechanisms for children and young people facing intolerable levels of stress and trauma.

In *The Body Keeps the Score*, Bessel van der Kolk (2014) outlines his theory of trauma, drawing upon extensive research and clinical practice. Van der Kolk suggests that trauma fundamentally alters both the brain and the body. It affects the limbic system which is responsible for our emotional and survival responses. Van der Kolk emphasises that trauma is not just a psychological issue, but is also a physiological one, where the body holds on to traumatic experiences, leading to a range of physical and emotional symptoms. This perspective has changed our understanding and treatment of trauma, highlighting the importance of integrating body-based therapies such as yoga and neurofeedback alongside more traditional psychological talking therapies. These approaches are considered in more detail in Chapters 7 and 8.

Understanding trauma and its effects on the brain is the first step towards supporting a child to manage and recover from trauma. Van der Kolk (2014) helpfully describes what is happening in the brain during a trauma response. Stress is our human response to overcoming danger and ensuring survival. The body's stress response worked well when our ancestors were faced with very real and immediate threats to their survival. However, that same life-saving, instinctive response that saved our ancestors from wild creatures is not so well adapted to the multiple forms of stress we encounter in modern life. Van Der Kolk uses stark imagery to describe how trauma affects the brain. He likened the amygdala to a **smoke detector** that constantly scans for danger. Van der Kolk describes the frontal lobes of the human brain, specifically the medial prefrontal cortex (MPFC), as a **watchtower**. The watchtower is constantly alert and can use rational thinking to decide whether there is a threat, and, if so, how great that threat is. Some people's smoke detectors will be more sensitive, perceiving a threat when there might not actually be one; they may also find it difficult to stop the alarm once it has started. This is especially true of those who are suffering from PTSD. Van der Kolk also compares the prefrontal cortex to a **cook** whose role is to plan and make decisions. When the smoke detector is not working efficiently, the cook becomes less effective, and this makes it hard to think clearly. He also describes the hippocampus as a **librarian** whose role is to organise our memories. When trauma is present, the hippocampus can become overwhelmed, leading to fragmented and intrusive memories of the original traumatic event.

This vivid imagery helps illustrate why trauma survivors often feel stuck in a state of fear and have difficulties processing their experiences. Finding accessible ways to help children (and parents) understand what is going on in the brain during a trauma response can be extremely helpful, and there are some great resources for doing this (see Additional resources section).

24 Supporting Children's Mental Health and Wellbeing

Young Minds (n.d.) suggest the following ways parents and practitioners can support a child who is experiencing trauma:

- Offer opportunities for them to talk
- Show that their feelings are understandable
- Help them feel safe and secure
- Reassure them
- Ask about what is making them feel this way
- Spend quality time doing things they enjoy
- Think together about what helps them cope
- Seek professional help.

The trauma response

Very often, what is going on in an individual's brain can affect how they behave in each situation. Walter Bradford Cannon (1915) first introduced the notion of *fight or flight* as an example of a trauma response to perceived danger. His work has subsequently been developed by other theorists to recognise a wider range of trauma responses, including *flop, freeze and fawn* (Walker 2013). Recognition of trauma responses can help practitioners make sense of children's actions reframing 'challenging behaviour' as the brain's rational response to a perceived threat. This can then be a game-changer in supporting the child to move forward. Consider the examples in Figure 2.2.

It would be all too easy to interpret each child's response in isolation and respond accordingly. However, seeing children's actions and reactions through a trauma awareness lens allows for a different interpretation and practitioner response. This is an idea we will return to throughout the book.

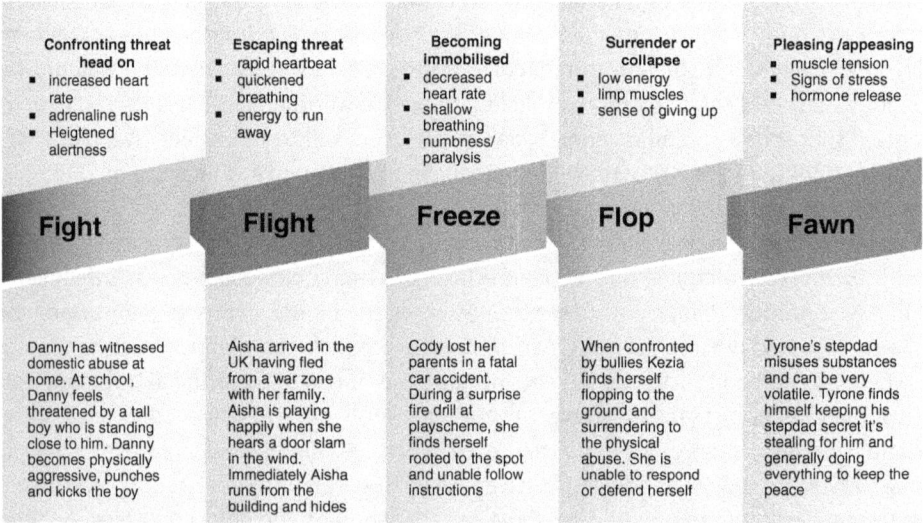

Figure 2.2 Stress response

Understanding adversity 25

REFLECTIVE TASK

Consider the following scenarios:

- Seven-year-old Jesse is at a class party when he suddenly becomes overwhelmed by loud noises. The situation becomes unbearable. As Jesse feels increasingly desperate, he seeks refuge in an empty room where he can feel safe.
- To avoid conflict, 11-year-old Lucy always agrees with whatever her friends want to do, even when it is something she feels uncomfortable with. When her friends suggest sneaking out of school early, Lucy hesitates, but ultimately goes along with it. She is terrified of their disapproval and seeks their acceptance by placating them at every turn.
- In soccer club, Raina is criticised by the coach for making a mistake. Overwhelmed by the criticism, she loses all motivation and stops participating, sits down in the field and refuses to continue.
- During a class presentation, 13-year-old Dan feels a wave of panic and his mind goes blank, even though it is a topic he knows well. He stands frozen, unable to move or speak as his body responds to the stress.
- Five-year-old Theo sees another child take his favourite toy without asking. Theo confronts the child, raising his voice and trying to snatch the toy back.

Which of the stress responses does each scenario represent? How might you intervene to support each child? What might you do preventively to prevent elevated stress for the children you work with?

Critical questions

- How helpful is the concept of ACEs in supporting your work with children and families? Are there any challenges to be aware of?
- Having explored the trauma responses of fight, flight, freeze, flop and fawn, can you think of examples from practice when you have seen these responses? How did you respond? How might you respond now in light of your reading?
- How does understanding how stress and trauma affect the brain help us to support children more effectively? How can you communicate this understanding to parents and children?

A focus on resilience

Resilience theory explores how individuals adapt and bounce back from adversity, stress and misfortune. It emphasises that the key factor is not the nature of the adversity itself, but how individuals respond to it. Resilience is seen as a dynamic process that involves positive adaptation within the context of significant adversity. Key elements of resilience theory include:

- **Adaptation and recovery** – resilience is the ability to maintain or regain mental health despite experiencing adversity
- **Dynamic process** – resilience is not a static trait but a process that can vary over time and across different situations
- **The influence of the environment** – actors such as supportive relationships, community resources and positive environments can enhance resilience.

(Moore, 2019)

It is important to note that there are many individual factors that affect a person's resilience. A person may show resilience in some areas of their lives, but not in others, and their resilience can change over time. Rutter (2012) emphasised that resilience is not just an individual trait but is also influenced by the environment and external factors. Garmezy (1992) highlighted that resilience is promoted in the presence of protective factors such as motivation, cognitive skills, autonomy and voice.

Researchers have found that there are many factors that contribute to individuals' resilience. These factors play a crucial role in fostering resilience, enabling individuals to thrive despite adversity and can include:

- Supportive relationships (Hart et al., 2007)
- Positive self-perception (Seligman, 2008)
- Effective coping skills such as problem solving, emotional regulation and stress management (Wilson, 2018)
- Community resources and social capital (Berkes & Ross, 2012)
- A sense of purpose supported by goals and aspirations (Lewis & Hill, 2021).

Angie Hart and her colleagues developed a resilience framework for children and young people (Boingboing.org, n.d). This framework provides a comprehensive approach, which is designed to promote resilience in individuals, particularly those who are facing significant adversity. The framework was drawn from research evidence, along with practical insights from practitioners working with disadvantaged children and families. The key components of the resilience framework include:

- Ensuring basic needs such as safety, health and a stable environment are met
- Fostering a strong sense of belonging and community
- Encouraging educational engagement and the development of problem-solving skills
- Building emotional regulation and stress management skills
- Promoting self-esteem, self-efficacy and a positive identity.

One of the main advantages of resilience theory, is that it positions resilience not as an innate trait that one either has or does not have, but as something that can be supported and developed. Within this context, parents and practitioners can use the framework to scaffold a child's resilience and to help the child make resilient moves (Aranda & Hart, 2015)

Understanding adversity 27

for themselves. (See Chapters 4 and 5 for more on resilience.) The practice vignette below explores how even children growing up in broadly similar circumstances may exhibit different levels of resilience.

 Practice vignette – a tale of three sisters

Amanda, Annette and Angela were born in the 1980s (so they are now in their forties.) Amanda is the oldest, Annette is the middle child (a year younger than Amanda) and Angela is two years younger than Annette.

The girls' dad died when Angela was just six months old. Their mum suffered severe depression and anxiety following her husband's death. The girls grew up in a very impoverished situation. There was often little food in the house, and both Annette and Amanda undertook a lot of household chores when their mum was unwell. Their attendance at school was sporadic and Annette became a school refuser. Angela and Annette both suffered from anxiety. However, Amanda continued to do well at school and went on to study at catering college. In her early twenties, Amanda did a part-time business studies degree at the local university. She now owns a large catering company and employs more than 100 staff. She owns her own home and has a family with her partner, Sam. She recently launched a training project for young people with mental health difficulties, for which she has won several awards.

Annette left school with no qualifications. She has had several short-term jobs, but her confidence remains low, and she has had long periods when she could not face leaving the house. She continues to care for her mother. Angela has had substance misuse issues, although she is not currently using drugs or alcohol. She has recently moved to a different area to get away from her peer group, which was not helping her in her quest to change her life. However, Angela is now working closely with her support worker to address some of her issues. She volunteers at the local community centre whilst pursuing a landscape gardening course.

Critical question

What factors might have contributed to the different outcomes for Amanda, Annette and Angela?

Hope as a superpower

When confronted with cases of challenging and multi-faceted adversity, it is crucial that, as practitioners, we see ourselves as purveyors and architects of hope (Prowle & Hodgkins, 2020). The *Cambridge Dictionary Online* (2023) defines hope as a belief or confidence that good things will happen in the future. Hockley (1993), writing in the context of palliative care, made the point that hope is more than wanting something to happen, it is something that engages our own agency. Hockley's work emphasises the importance of hope in people who are seriously ill, the 'will to live' being the ultimate expression of personal hope.

Snyder et al. (2000) argue that there are three important aspects to hope:

- **Goals** - focused thought to identify goals in life
- **Pathways** - strategies developed to achieve goals
- **Agency** - self-belief and motivation to make the effort required to reach these goals.

They argue that hopeful people are those who can establish their own clear goals, devise ways to meet these goals and be able to persevere, even when things become difficult. If one of these three components is missing, then a person will lose their sense of hope. This presents a helpful approach for practitioners seeking to engage children and families with hope. Throughout this book, hope is a theme that keeps recurring, and we will explore in more detail how practitioners can harness their own hope for families facing adversity, and, more importantly, help to stir and inspire that same hope in those they work with.

Conclusion

This chapter has dealt with complex issues and emotionally challenging material. There is compelling evidence that many children and young people are challenged by multiple adversities. There is also a growing evidence base that without effective intervention, adversity can have lasting and profound impacts, leading to sub-optimal outcomes across the life course. The broader and deeper those adversities are, and the longer they last, the more they become compounded making it even more difficult to change. However, there is also evidence that an attuned practitioner (see Chapter 10), working in a strength-based way, focusing on resilience and modelling hope can make a real difference and support children to better outcomes. Chapters 4-9 explore specific approaches that can be applied to supporting children and families to achieve positive outcomes.

Adversity: key points

- Whilst adversity is an inevitable part of life, multiple adversities can accumulate and affect all parts of a child's life, making it more difficult for them to achieve positive outcomes.
- Trauma is a response to distressing events. Trauma is highly individual and although individuals may experience similar events or adversities, people respond to them differently for a range of reasons including personality traits, previous life experiences and the support around them.
- What is happening within the brain largely determines our trauma response. Understanding how the brain responds in stressful situations is helpful in enabling us to respond appropriately.
- Children and families can be supported to develop resilience in the face of adversity.

ADDITIONAL RESOURCES

- Boingboing.org – Boingboing is a multi-faceted resilience website, with a range of helpful resilience resources. The website "aims to model and promote resilience research and practice that challenges social inequalities, in pursuit of a loving, fun and fair world where individuals from all walks of life are valued and respected".

- Van der Kolk (2014) *The body keeps the score* – Bessel Van der Kolk is a Dutch psychiatrist who explores the effects of trauma on mind and body. The book draws on case files to consider a range of therapeutic approaches. There is a strong focus on resilience and wellbeing.

- Webb *et al.* (2014) *Living with adversity: a qualitative study of families with multiple and complex needs* – The research presented in this report was jointly conducted by Barnardo's, NSPCC NI, the National Children's Bureau (NCB NI) and the Queen's University of Belfast (QUB). Whilst it focuses on Northern Ireland, it has wider application. This report presents a range of research evidence and, most importantly, gives a voice to families directly experiencing multiple problems.

- www.beaconhouse.org.uk – There are a range of free resources related to trauma that have been developed for parents and practitioners on this website.

References

Aranda, K. and Hart, A., (2015) Resilient moves: tinkering with practice theory to generate new ways of thinking about using resilience. *Health*, 19(4), pp. 355–371.

Bellis, M.A., Ashton, K., Hughes, K., Ford, K.J., Bishop, J. and Paranjothy S. (2015) Adverse childhood experiences and their impact on health-harming behaviours in the Welsh adult population. Cardiff: Public Health Wales.

Bellis, M.A., Lowey, H., Leckenby, N., Hughes, K. and Harrison, D. (2014) Adverse childhood experiences: retrospective study to determine their impact on adult health behaviours and health outcomes in a UK population. *Journal of Public Health*, 36(1), pp. 81–91.

Bellis, M.A. Hughes, K., Ford, K., Rodriguez, G.R., Sethi, D. and Passmore, J. (2019) Life course health consequences and associated annual costs of adverse childhood experiences across Europe and North America: a systematic review and meta-analysis. *Lancet Public Health*, 4(10), pp. e517–e528.

Berkes, F. and Ross, H. (2012) Community resilience: toward an integrated approach. *Society & Natural Resources*, 26(1), pp. 5–20. doi:10.1080/08941920.2012.736605.

Boingboing.org (n.d.) Available at: https://www.boingboing.org.uk (Accessed 29 January 2025).

Bronfenbrenner, U. (1979) *The ecology of human development: experiments by nature and design*. Cambridge, MA: Harvard University Press.

Cannon, W.B. (1915) *Bodily changes in pain, hunger, fear, and rage*. New York: Appleton-Century-Crofts.

Cambridge Dictionary Online. Available at: https://dictionary.cambridge.org/dictionary/english-french (Accessed 20 September 2024).

Centre on the Developing Child, Harvard University. (2024) *A guide to toxic stress*. Available at: https://developingchild.harvard.edu/guide/a-guide-to-toxic-stress (Accessed 17 August 2024).

ComplexTrauma.org (n.d.) Available at: https://www.complextrauma.org/complex-trauma/complex-trauma-what-is-it-and-how-does-it-affect-people (Accessed 1 September 2024).

Felitti, V.J., Anda, R.F., Nordenberg, D., Williamson, D.F., Spitz, A.M., Edwards, V. and Marks, J.S. (1998) Relationship of childhood abuse and household dysfunction to many of the leading causes of death in adults: the Adverse Childhood Experiences (ACE) Study. *American Journal of Preventive Medicine*, 14(4), pp. 245-258.

Friedman, B.D. and Allen, K.N. (2011) Systems theory. *Theory & Practice in Clinical Social Work*, 2(3), pp. 3-20.

Garmezy, N. (1991) Resiliency and vulnerability to adverse developmental outcomes associated with poverty, *The American Behavioural Scientist*, 34, 416.

Hart, A., Blincow, D. and Thomas, H. (2007) *Resilient therapy: Working with children and families*. Hove: Routledge.

Hart, A., Gagnon, E., Eryigit-Madzwamuse, S., Cameron, J., Aranda, K., Rathbone, A. and Heaver, B. (2016) Uniting resilience research and practice with an inequalities approach. *Sage Open*, 6(4), p. 2158244016682477.

Hartas, D. (2019) Assessing the foundational studies on adverse childhood experiences, *Social Policy and Society*, 18(3), pp. 435-443.

Hockley, J. (1993) The concept of hope and the will to live, *Palliative Medicine*, 7(3), pp. 181-186.

Hodgkins, A. and Prowle, A. (2023) *Strength-based practice with children and families*. St Albans: Critical Publishing.

Hood, R., Goldacre, A., Webb, C., Bywaters, P., Gorin, S. and Clements, K. (2021) Beyond the toxic trio: exploring demand typologies in children's social care, *British Journal of Social Work*, 51(6), pp. 1942-1962.

Keller, H., (1903) *Optimism: an essay*. New York: C. Y. Crowell and Company.

Lester, S., Khatwa, M. and Sutcliffe, K. (2020) Service needs of young people affected by adverse childhood experiences (ACEs): a systematic review of UK qualitative evidence, *Children and Youth Services Review*, 118, p. 105429.

Lewis, N.A. and Hill, P.L. (2021) Sense of purpose promotes resilience to cognitive deficits attributable to depressive symptoms, *Frontiers in Psychology*, 12, p. 698109.

Lewis, S.J., Arseneault, L., Caspi, A., Fisher, H.L., Matthews, T., Moffitt, T.E., Odgers, C.L., Stahl, D., Teng, J.Y. and Danese, A. (2019) The epidemiology of trauma and post-traumatic stress disorder in a representative cohort of young people in England and Wales, *The Lancet Psychiatry*, 6(3), pp. 247-256.

Maslow, A.H. (1954) The instinctoid nature of basic needs. *Journal of Personality*, 22, 326-347.

Merriam Webster Dictionary (2002) Available at: https://www.merriam-webster.com.

Merrick, M.T., Ford, D.C., Ports, K.A. *et al.* (2019) Vital signs: estimated proportion of adult health problems attributable to adverse childhood experiences and implications for prevention – 25 states, 2015-2017. *Morbidity and Mortality Weekly Report*, 68(44):, pp. 999-1005. doi:http://dx.doi.org/10.15585/mmwr.mm6844e1 (Accessed 16 September 2024).

Moore, C. (2019) Resilience theory: a summary of the research. Available at https://positivepsychology.com/resilience-theory (Accessed 17 September 2024).

Prowle, A. and Hodgkins, A. (2020) *Making a difference with children and families: re-imagining the role of the practitioner*. London: Bloomsbury Publishing.

Prowle, A. and Musgrave, J. (2018) Utilising strengths in families and communities to support children's learning and wellbeing, in *Pedagogies for leading practice* (), Abingdon: Routledge, pp. 125-141.

Rankin, J. and Regan, S. (2004) Meeting complex needs in social care. *Housing, Care, and Support*, 7(3), pp. 4-8.

Rutter, M. (2012) Resilience as a dynamic concept. *Development and Psychopathology*, 24(2), pp. 335-344.

Saleeby, D. (1996) The strengths perspective in social work practice: extensions and cautions. *Social Work*, 41(3), pp. 296-305.

Schofield, T.J., Donnellan, M.B., Merrick, M.T., Ports, K.A., Klevens, J. and Leeb, R. (2018) Intergenerational continuity in adverse childhood experiences and rural community environments. *American Journal of Public Health*, 108(9), pp. 1148-1152. doi: https://doi.org/10.2105/AJPH.2018.304598.

Schofield, T.J, Lee, R.D. and Merrick, M.T. (2013) Safe, stable, nurturing relationships as a moderator of intergenerational continuity of child maltreatment: a meta-analysis. *Journal of Adolescent Health*, 53(4 Suppl.), S32-38. doi: https://doi.org/10.1016/j.jadohealth.2013.05.004.

Seligman, M.E. (2008) Positive health. *Applied Psychology*, 57, pp. 3-18.

Skinner, G.C., Bywaters, P.W., Bilson, A., Duschinsky, R., Clements, K. and Hutchinson, D. (2021) The 'toxic trio' (domestic violence, substance misuse and mental ill-health): how good is the evidence base? *Children and Youth Services Review*, 120(Jan.), pp. 105-678.

Snyder, C.R., Ilardi, S.S., Cheavens, J., Michael, S.T., Yamhure, L. and Sympson, S. (2000) The role of hope in cognitive-behaviour therapies. *Cognitive Therapy and Research*, 24, pp. 747-762.

Springs, F. and Friedrich, W.N. (1992) Health risk behaviours and medical sequelae of childhood sexual abuse. *Mayo Clinic Proceedings*, 67(6), pp. 527–532.

Van der Kolk, B.A. (2014) *The body keeps the score: mind, brain, and body in the transformation of trauma*. London: Penguin.

Wadsworth, M.E. (2015) Development of maladaptive coping: a functional adaptation to chronic, uncontrollable stress. *Child Development Perspectives*, 9(2), pp. 96–100.

Walker, P. (2013) *Complex PTSD: from surviving to thriving: a guide and map for recovering from childhood trauma*. Gloucester: CreateSpace.

Wilson, G.A. (2018) "Constructive tensions" in resilience research: critical reflections from a human geography perspective, *The Geographical Journal*, 184(1), pp. 89–99.

Young Minds Trauma. Trauma and mental health : a guide for parents. Available at: https://www.youngminds.org.uk/parent/parents-a-z-mental-health-guide/trauma (Accessed 19 September 2024).

3
Supporting the holistic needs of children and families

Introduction

Would you rather be rich but have no one to love you, or be poor and loved? Few people would choose money over relationships, highlighting their huge significance to our wellbeing. In this chapter we analyse how attachment relates to development, particularly when working with trauma-experienced children and families. We use the Circles of Security programme to illustrate what this looks like in practice, going beyond an instrumental key person approach. Pestalozzi's Head, Heart and Hands is outlined as a tool to help us focus on holistic wellbeing, as well as fostering an emotionally safe and enabling environment that meets children's psychological needs.

The importance of sensitive and attuned relationships

'Attachment' is the word used to define an emotionally restorative relationship between people, or as John Bowlby put it, a "lasting psychological connectedness between human beings" (1969, p.194). In the 1940s Bowlby was commissioned by the World Health Organisation (WHO) to study the cause of 'maladjustment' in boys. A common factor was a poor or non-existent maternal relationship. Bowlby knew about studies conducted by Harlow with baby rhesus monkeys who, when frightened, chose to cling to a soft, comforting 'mother' rather than a wire, feeding 'mother'. Bowlby also studied Lorenz's work on imprinting that suggested attachment was biologically innate (at least in ducklings). Based on these conclusions, he proposed that attachment was vital to survival, which was very radical at the time.

Others later extended Bowlby's attachment theory, particularly Mary Ainsworth, who stressed the importance of someone (not necessarily the child's mother) to act as a "secure base", providing a "safe haven" when the child was distressed. Ainsworth and Bell devised an assessment technique called The Strange Situation (1970) that categorised children's attachment patterns as either *secure* or *insecure* (*avoidant* or *ambivalent*). Later, working with her husband, Erik Hesse, a fourth category, *disorganised*, was added.

Although these findings might seem obvious, we should not presume that attachment is simple; the complexities arising from insecure attachments cannot be overstated. Goleman (1996) draws on research by LeDoux who proposed that the foundations of emotional life are significantly impacted by the responses of caregivers in the early years and held in the amygdala, the section of the brain that processes emotions, such as fear, fight or flight and memory. These relational experiences formed as infants are suppressed in the subconscious. Golman refers to these as "emotional memories" (Goleman, 1996, p.22) because they are formed before the child can articulate experiences through language. Emotional memories can be triggered seemingly without cause, as Goleman explains,

> One reason we can be so baffled by our emotional outbursts, then, is that they often date from a time when we did not yet have the words for comprehending events. We may have the chaotic feelings, but not the words for the memories that formed them.
>
> (Goleman, 1996, p.22)

This creates difficulties at a time when children's social and emotional development is being constructed.

Insecurely attached children frequently have difficulty relating to others as they progress through adolescence into adulthood, rejecting people and avoiding situations where feelings of anxiety and vulnerability may resurface. This can lead to them becoming emotionally unavailable and distrustful of others, as the fight or flight hormone epinephrine, or adrenaline, is released into the bloodstream (Pietromonaco & Powers, 2015). In contrast, children with a secure attachment learn to regulate their emotions, manage anxiety, develop social and emotional skills and respond well to challenge (Bergin & Bergin, 2009). It is estimated that at least one third of children have an insecure attachment (Bergin & Bergin, 2009).

> **REFLECTIVE TASK**
>
> There are various reasons why children develop insecure attachments. Use the table below to consider possible reasons. Can you think of any other risk factors?

Table 3.1 Potential risk factors of insecure attachments between child and parent/caregiver

Risk factors of insecure attachment between child and parent/caregiver	Possible reasons
Poverty	
Parental mental health problems	
Neglect and other abuse	
Parental substance abuse	
Premature birth	
Multiple siblings	
Family bereavement	
'Surprise' baby	

Attachment sabotaging

The logical solution to supporting a child with an insecure attachment style is to provide the consistent, loving responses they were denied. Sadly, as a result of the internalisation of negative messages, for example, that they are 'naughty' or 'bad' and that caregivers are unpredictable, children can become conditioned to believe that they are unworthy of love.

Although confusing and disturbing these feelings are familiar, and children may subconsciously try to recreate an environment where they feel vulnerable and unloved. After seemingly making progress in building a trusting relationship with a caring new adult, insecurely attached children may regress to wetting or soiling themselves. This situation, with both the associated smells and feeling of shame, is bizarrely comforting at the same time as it is reassuringly familiar and predictable (Naish et al., 2023, p.313).

Just as children may recreate this familiar sensory environment, they may also replicate a familiar emotional environment. Accustomed to chaos and disappointment, when rewarded with kindness by a new caregiver the child may unwittingly self-sabotage the attachment by becoming violent, destroying objects and being verbally abusive (Naish et al., 2023, p.269). From the child's perspective the loving response is unexpected and goes against their internal working model as being unworthy of love. To protect themselves from rejection, insecurely attached children will sometimes reject the caregiver before they are rejected. This relationship sabotaging cycle frequently persists throughout the child's life (Slade, 2019). Thankfully, however, the cycle is reversible (Bergin & Bergin, 2009; Black, 2019) and well-informed caregivers and professionals can be hugely influential in addressing this.

Understanding behaviour as communication

Teachers, with the pressure to teach and assess knowledge and skills, may be unaware that children's behaviour is a reflection of their mental and emotional state, often connected to their early attachment experiences (Wright, 2009). When children 'misbehave' it is often a "highly emotional experience" for both the child and the teacher (Wright, 2009, p.286). By remembering that the child probably has an ambivalent attachment style and is communicating their anxiety, vulnerability and fear of abandonment caused by having their needs met only sporadically, teachers and other professionals can view children's behaviour objectively, rather than personally. The child is torn between internal competing demands; the need for love and belonging, juxtaposed with the need to protect their inner self from anticipated hurt and disappointment, resulting in oppositional behaviour (Wright, 2009). If adults are unaware of the potential root causes of the behaviour, there is a danger of aggression escalating on both sides.

Conversely, behaviour that is too compliant or independent should not be overlooked. A child who has developed an internal working model that caregivers are unpredictable can compensate by becoming overly self-sufficient. In the longer term this can also affect their ability to maintain fulfilling relationships (Morris, 2015). If children are to learn that adults can be trusted, adults must show that they are strong enough to act as a container for the child's feelings of anxiety and vulnerability (Casement, 1985) (see Chapter 5 for more on containment).

A constant reflective stance must be maintained, however, to avoid adopting a reductionist view of the child and subconsciously framing them as a 'victim' or 'broken'. This may lead to 'othering' or perhaps treating them as what Foucault termed "cases" to be trained, corrected, classified, normalised or excluded (Foucault, 1977, p.191). In acknowledging that social factors affect children's behaviour, we would do well to remember that children are individuals and not merely the sum of their circumstances.

Attention seeking versus attachment needing

Insecurely attached children can act in 'challenging' ways, demanding to be seen and heard. This is often referred to as 'attention seeking behaviour'. Cooper (1999) proposes that society, particularly schools, struggles to know how to respond to these 'challenging' children. The instinct might be to demonstrate disapproval through the withholding of eye contact, smiles and other positively affirming gestures in the hope that children will be punished into conformity. The withdrawal of emotional intimacy however, "psychologically distances the child from caregivers and diminishes possibilities for any 'human' connection that the child may be seeking" (Wright, 2009, p.287).

Consider the subliminal messages relayed by our language use; in labelling children as 'attention seeking', the blame is situated within the child rather than what is causing the behaviour. Ignoring the behaviour and withdrawing approval can escalate tensions and the child may become increasingly demanding to highlight their distress, or their expectations that adults are inconsistent and emotionally unavailable are confirmed. As Bowlby noted, the child views themselves as not only "unwanted, but unwantable" (Bowlby, 1973, p.204). Looking for the cause of the behaviour requires applying professional emotional discipline, refraining from indulging in offence taking and maintaining an overall perspective.

Once behaviour is understood as communicating a need caregivers can reassure children that they are not forgotten (Geddes, 2017), perhaps by offering regular, quality connection time. This may be engaging with them as soon as the child and caregiver come together, either in an activity that involves just the two of them, or a casual chat about how their day has been (Naish *et al.*, 2023).

Circles of Security

Building on attachment theory Circles of Security is an intervention that supports children's emotional development (Huber *et al.*, 2018). Taking a strengths-based approach, caregivers learn to build on what has already been accomplished and assets or interests the child has, rather than the problems (Powell *et al.*, 2014). As Baron *et al.* explain focusing on what is 'strong' and not what is 'wrong' can completely change the discourse (Baron *et al.*, 2019, p.93).

A central part of the Circles of Security intervention is a graphic illustrating the key components of the intervention (Maxwell *et al.*, 2021, p.1125).

A circle is presented with children's basic needs explored at different times. Firstly, "going out on the circle", then, "coming in on the circle" and, finally, "hands on the circle".

The *going out* part of the graphic relates to children's bids to explore the world independently. This is encouraged, with the child knowing that the caregiver is a *secure base*, watching their adventures from a distance, but still within reach, providing any help necessary and even participating if invited. This enables the child to become competent and autonomous.

When children are *"coming in"*, perhaps upset, tired or anxious, they need the caregiver to fill their emotional cup by being a *safe haven*, soothing, empathising and showing pleasure at their return (Huber et al., 2018).

Throughout the cycle the caregiver has three main roles:

1. To be emotionally strong and available
2. To flexibly offer warmth and support, secure boundaries, supervision and direction
3. To follow the child's lead but be ready to "actively intervene", i.e. step in when the child is not managing risk safely, offer solutions to difficult situations and/or provide "behavioural and emotional containment" (Huber et al., 2018, p.2).

The adults are the *"hands on the circle"*, reassuringly in charge, attuned to know when to allow the child to lead and when to make appropriate interventions. In essence they should be "bigger and stronger, wiser and kind" (Marvin et al., 2002, p.110).

When the adult has an insecure attachment

A successful Circle of Security depends upon a sensitive caregiver. Remembering, however, that at least one third of children have an insecure attachment (Bergin & Bergin, 2009) it is likely that many have become adults with unresolved attachment needs themselves. The Circles of Security programme encourages caregivers to be alert to any subconscious unmet need from their own experience of being parented. The risk is that when the child needs the adult to rise above feelings of irritation or even aggression the adults' unmet need is triggered by the child's behaviour, overwhelms them and the adult struggles to be "bigger and stronger, wiser and kind" (Marvin et al., 2002, p.110). In Circles of Security this is referred to as "shark music". If the caregiver acts defensively the danger is that the child withholds their emotions and mistrust can develop. When the child involuntarily encounters the adult's unmet attachment needs their circle of security is compromised, described as "limited circles, limited hands" (Huber et al., 2018, p.3). A key part of the Circle of Security programme involves working with the caregiver to identify and resolve any potential issues before it negatively affects their relationship with the child ("the linchpin") (Huber et al., 2018, p.3).

 Case study: Circle of Security; *Time in*

The following case study is adapted from the Circles of Security website. It illustrates that when adults are bigger and stronger, wiser and kind as they hold boundaries, the child feels safe, supported and able to explore the world from a secure base.

> *Amelia, a single mother of two-year-old Malik, attended a Circle of Security parenting class because she was struggling with Malik's behaviour. Amelia recognised the need to set boundaries with Malik and had adopted a 'time out' approach, making him stay in his room when he misbehaved. Malik would initially protest angrily, and then sob himself to*

sleep. Although Amelia felt pleased that she was setting boundaries, she also felt anxious and guilty that Malik was left alone when he was so upset.

Amelia and Malik worked with the facilitator, Connie, who was also a licensed mental health counsellor and knew Amelia well. Connie asked Amelia if she wanted to learn to set boundaries in a bigger and stronger, wiser and kind way, and Amelia agreed. Connie directed Amelia to take Malik to an area away from the others attending the session – Malik resisted, shouting and kicking Ameila. Connie encouraged Amelia to respond in a soothing manner and gently rub Malik's back. Connie gave a verbal commentary, for example, "you're having a tough day" and "it's hard when you feel so angry".

Although Malik continued to struggle Ameila held him lightly, but with strength. Even when Malik became aggressive, she calmly held his arms, while Connie reminded him to use gentle hands with his mother. Soon Malik's protests and break away attempts escalated, leaving Amelia feeling overwhelmed. Connie encouraged Amelia to persist with her gentle approach because although he was pulling away this was when Malik needed her most.

Before long Malik began to cry and turned towards Amelia for a hug, who stroked his hair and held him close. After a few minutes, Malik faced Amelia and smiled, asking her for help with his shoes. He then went to play with the other children.

Tearfully Amelia told Connie that that had never happened before, but that it had felt good. Connie praised Amelia on being consistent, explaining that Malik needed her to contain his big emotions with her strong body, gentle hands and soothing voice. Connie explained that they had gone through a relationship repair, after the break down when Amelia had initiated the boundary. When Malik learned that Amelia could hold the boundary and his emotions, he relaxed and leaned on her, fixing the rupture in their relationship.

(Adapted from *Time In, a true-life example*, The Circle of Security International, 2022)

Critical questions

1. In what ways was Amelia conflicted in her relationship with Malik?
2. How would you describe the relationship between Connie and Amelia?
3. How significant was Amelia's indication that she was ready to learn and change? Why?
4. What are the pros and cons of adopting a *time in* mindset?
5. What did Malik need from Amelia and how did she meet these needs?

Beyond the key person

The Early Years Foundation Stage Statutory Framework (Department for Education, 2023, p.28), the English framework for early years practitioners, states that all children must be designated a key person, responsible for ensuring that the care offered is appropriate for the child's individual needs, helping them settle in, building a relationship with the child and their family and accessing additional support services, if necessary. An attachment style relationship built on affection and commitment is implicit (Elfer *et al.*, 2003), however, it is arguably impossible to legislate for relationships, leading many key persons to assume a more instrumental approach, for example, focusing on undertaking personal care tasks and updating developmental progress records.

Noddings argues that caregivers, particularly educators, have a duty to go beyond this technician approach. Teachers and practitioners have a responsibility not only to teach children curriculum content, but to care "in a way that contributes to the creation of caring, competent, loving and lovable people" (Noddings, 1995, p.24). She explains that to be effective, educators must consider *how they care* as well as *what they do*, highlighting the difference between assuming a duty of care and an ethic of care. It is entirely possible to 'care give' without feeling any sense of caring towards the recipient (Kawamura & Eisler, 2013).

Those who care for children in the absence of a parent have a legal responsibility to act *in loco parentis*, to act in the place of a parent. Taking a similar approach to Noddings, Van Manen (1991) urges educators to remember the relational aspect of their *in loco parentis* responsibility, writing,

> What is relevant for the relation between parents and children may be informative for the pedagogical relation between teachers and students. As schools and other childcare institutions have taken on more and more responsibilities previously dealt with within the family, professional educations need to become more reflective about what in loco parentis entails.
>
> (Van Manen, 1991, p.5)

This might include offering routines and consistency which build children's sense of identity and self-worth. It may also be listening in a non-judgemental way, and fostering "responsible self-awareness, a personal sense of direction and how one ought to deal with life" (Van Manen, 1991, p.86). The practice vignette below explores how practitioners can support children's conflict resolution and model positive interactions.

 Practice vignette

Tara is an early career teacher working in an area of high social and economic deprivation. Many of the children belong to hybrid families, frequently changing due to parental separation and divorce, re-marriage and new relationships. One break-time two children in Tara's class come into the classroom complaining that the other has acted unfairly. The situation has escalated, and the two former friends cannot see one another's perspective; both are emotional and defiant.

Tara's instinct is to send them back into the playground with a '"stop being silly" response, but a more experienced teacher encounters the children first. The teacher takes a few moments to de-escalate the situation by listening carefully to both sides asking, "Is that everything?" after each child has finished speaking. Both children explain the situation from their perspective. The teacher makes reflective statements such as, "OK, I see. So, you thought she didn't want to be your friend any more …?" After both children have had the

Supporting the holistic needs of children & families 39

opportunity to talk the teacher asks what they would like to happen now and helps them repair their relationship and then uses humour to lighten the mood and enable re-bonding.

After the children have gone Tara speaks with the teacher about why they got involved in the children's squabble. The teacher explains that these children may not have the negotiation skills to move forward when relationships become stuck because of a lack of positive conflict resolution role models in their family homes. Having these skills cultivated at school is as important as any curriculum learning.

Tara takes this on board and makes a conscious effort to model respectful relationships with everyone in the school community.

Critical question

Do you agree that modelling good relationships and supporting children's conflict resolution skills is as important as curriculum learning? Why?

Holistic wellbeing

To be a positive role model who understands that educating children is for life, not only for exams, practitioners, teachers and caregivers should take a holistic approach to children's development. Traditionally holistic development has included children's physical, intellectual, emotional, social and spiritual development (PIESS). This tradition moved away from narrowly focusing on cognitive ability and assessment preparation, acknowledging that learning cannot be compartmentalised because each area impacts on another (Bruce, 1987). There is, however, a danger that holistic development is simplified to become part of a skills-based process whereby practitioners measure children's progress against predetermined outcomes; viewed through a PIESS lens in which holistic wellbeing is considered a precursor to learning and development. The focus is still on attainment, with an emphasis on curriculum delivery rather than the children's holistic lives.

International research undertaken by educator and theorist Barbara Rogoff showing that children learn by participating in their culture has widened our understanding of holistic learning and development. Eavesdropping on adult conversations, hearing stories about ancestors, being teased, praised, noting attitudes towards education, spirituality, acceptable behaviour (for example, eye contact and silence) social routines, personal space and chores are all absorbed by children. They become enculturated by assimilating the aspirations and hidden values in their culture, working out the "scripts" of everyday life through their play and "intent community participation" (Rogoff, 2003, p.298). Communities have differing views on what a "good life" looks like and both societal conditions and traditions arguably have a greater impact on children's development than direct, formal instruction (Hedegaard, 2009).

Taking a genuinely holistic approach to working with children and families involves appreciating "the whole child, body, mind, feelings, spirit and creativity. Crucially, the child is seen as a social being, connected to others and at the same time with their own distinctive experiences and knowledge" (Petrie *et al.*, 2008, p.3). This holistic, social pedagogical view of the child encourages caregivers to take a life world orientation approach, considering "a person's personality, strengths, likes, dislikes, their extended family and friends, culture, religion, place of upbringing and significant events in their lives" (Kaska, 2015, p.43).

It is human nature for our behaviour to be guided by our own values and successfully responding to the holistic child demands "disciplining our character" (Stobbs, 2023, p.9). A survivor of concentration camps and later an influential psychiatrist-author Viktor E. Frankl wrote about how some prisoners, when placed in positions of authority gave preferential treatment to their friends. Withholding judgement Frankl reflected, "No man should judge unless he asks himself in absolute honesty whether in a similar situation, he might not have done the same" (Frankl, 1959, p.26).

Similarly, albeit on a lesser scale, we might be critical of a friend's choices ("I would never eat a whole family bar of chocolate in an evening"), but we are thinking of what *we* would do, with our upbringing and experiences, the values and traditions that we have absorbed. Instead of instinctively condemning people for their actions we should pause and consider the deeper message being communicated. When we are curious rather than disapproving, appreciating that any hurtful behaviour is not personal, we can maintain composure.

Critical questions

- What is the danger of focusing on PIESS when considering holistic development?
- How would you define learning by 'enculturation'?
- Can you think of an example in your own life?
- How does understanding the holistic nature of children's learning and taking a life world orientation help us when working with children and families?
- Why should we avoid making judgements about others based on our own values and experiences?

Implications for frontline practitioners seeking to create emotionally safe and nurturing environments

Julia Hancock (2018) wrote about her journey from banker to educator, reflecting that although she was a head teacher, she was also a "heart teacher", using her acquired professionalism to represent the best interests of her school community (the head), whilst equally feeling empathy for individuals experiencing troubling situations (the heart) (Hancock, 2018, p.79). The concept of a "heart teacher" is inspirational, but should perhaps include a third element, a "hands" teacher, the practical application of theory, combined with empathy as outlined by Pestalozzi's Head, Heart, Hands model (Silber, 1965) where the whole self is engaged when working with children and families.

The model is most easily understood when we consider what happens when one of the three elements is missing.

Supporting the holistic needs of children & families 41

Table 3.2 Head, Heart and Hands, what's missing?

Elements	Outcome
Head + Heart =	A knowledgeable and empathetic response but no action (nothing gets done)
Head + Hands =	A knowledgeable and practical response but no empathy (going through the motions)
Heart + Hands =	Action driven by empathy, but not informed by theory, experience and/or knowledge (it felt like the right thing to do, no one knows why')
Head + Heart + Hands =	A response informed by theory, experience and knowledge, feelings of empathy, combined with the practical skills to follow through.

> **REFLECTIVE TASK**
>
> In the following situations reflect on which of the elements Head, Heart, Hands model you would draw on.

Table 3.3 Head, Heart or Hands; what does each situation call for?

Situation	Head, Heart or Hands?
Reading a book	
Painting	
Doing a jigsaw	
Writing a report	
Cooking	
Bowling	
Putting a plaster on a child's injury	
Asking why a child has been absent from school	
Responding to a child who has knocked all the art materials off the desk	

You may have found yourself thinking, 'it depends on ...' which is just the right perspective to take! In adopting a holistic approach, we recognise that there are no straightforward answers or flow charts telling us how to respond. Using our Head, Heart and Hands in each unique family context is arguably professionalism in its highest form. Doing the right thing as well as doing things right (Munro, 2010) takes courage, acting in the moment according to your values. There is no toolkit, just yourself.

Meeting children's psychological needs

Theories are valuable because they help us understand why something might have happened and predict what might happen in the future. One theory that considers human motivation is Maslow's Hierarchy of Needs (1943). He proposed that before people could enjoy being creative or intellectually stimulated, their basic needs had to be met, for example,

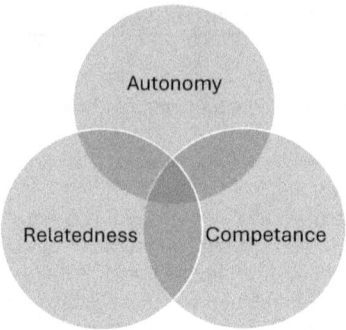

Figure 3.1 The three psychological needs

food, sleep and safety. This formulation is instinctively relatable when working with children; we know that they will struggle to concentrate if they are thinking about how hungry they are.

A theory by Deci and Ryan (2000, 2002) adds to that of Maslow (see Chapter 5 for more on this). Based on years of research into human motivation they identified why people do what they do and developed Self-Determination Theory, which proposes that everyone, including children, has three innate, basic psychological needs. If we understand and cultivate these, we can create an emotionally safe, empowering and nurturing environment. The three needs are: relatedness (I belong), competence (I can) and autonomy (I can be me) (Morris, 2015) (see Figure 3.1).

What do each of the components mean?

Relatedness – you feel unconditionally loved and cared for by your group, and vice versa.
Competence – what is asked of you is pitched at the right level for you to develop, grow and learn. It is neither too hard nor too easy.
Autonomy – you feel in control of your life and able to act according to your values and beliefs.
> The model proposes that if one or more of the three needs are unmet, people try to cope by putting up defences, acting aggressively, experiencing anxiety or responding in their personal self-interest. As when considering the Head, Heart, Hands model, it can help our understanding to imagine what life would be like if each of the components were absent. Let's look at each in turn.

Relatedness – Consider all the groups or associations to which you belong. Now imagine not having any of these relationships, how would this impact on your esteem and sense of identity? Have you ever felt like an outsider? Why did you feel this way? How did you react? Imagine, for example, going to support your favourite team and inadvertently finding yourself sitting in the away team section.
Competence – Have you ever been asked to do something that is too difficult? Too easy? Or been offered multiple options? This is deeply frustrating and if sustained for an extended period there is a danger of internalised behaviour developing, such as panic attacks, self-harm and anxiety.

Autonomy – Have you ever felt powerless? Perhaps when using public transport and a service is cancelled. People respond in different ways in the face of disempowerment – some may try to re-assert their power by becoming aggressive, others become despondent at not being listened to. If you have a personal relationship with the person making the announcement, however, does this change the reaction? What does this show about the importance of relationships?

When contemplating children's motivations and needs, however, we might add another element, that of fun! Although learning is not always fun or entertaining (Katz & Chard, 2000) fun is often hugely motivating (Hewitson, 2021). This does not mean telling endless jokes or being ridiculously silly, rather, it involves being light-hearted, seeing the funny side of things and being spontaneous. Having fun and being funny contributes to the three psychological needs – it can bring people together (relatedness), take the sting out of having no choice about a task (autonomy) and reduce anxiety when the risk of failure seems overwhelming (competence).

What does it mean to you?

Finally, don't ask why

When things go wrong, and children make mistakes it is tempting to ask them why they acted the way they did. This is not usually because we are giving the child an opportunity to respond but because we want to reprimand them. If they were able to articulate why they did what they did (for example, "Because I was remembering that my dad has left, and his girlfriend is having a baby, and I felt sad and alone …") then we might learn something about the child's world that would enable us to support them rather than shame them (Van Manen, 1991).

Children who have experienced trauma and inconsistent caregiving may not understand cause and effect (causality), which means they cannot logically compute the natural consequences of their behaviour. This gap in development means that punishments are often ineffective because they have not learned that when they do X, Y will happen (Naish *et al.*, 2023). What is more effective is waiting until the heat has gone from the moment, and then explaining to the child what they did and what they should do next time (Naish *et al.*, 2023).

Conclusion

In this chapter we began by exploring the importance of attachment on wellbeing and the critical need for developing sensitive and attuned relationships. We highlighted that children who have suffered trauma or neglect may have had experiences that impact on their ability to relate to others. This might cause them to sabotage these relationships as a way of communicating a need for secure boundaries and testing your commitment to them. The Circles of Security programme was discussed as an example of attachment-based care, and we noted the importance of reflecting on our own attachment style before intervening. To help us understand the best way to help children we must non-judgementally consider the whole child. Using the concept of life world orientation reminds us that before we intervene, we must try to understand the world from their perspective. Pestalozzi's Head, Heart, Hands is a useful tool when focusing on holistic wellbeing, ensuring that our practice is intentional and informed. Finally, once we have these factors in place we can focus on meeting children and families' three innate, basic psychological needs and create emotionally safe and enabling environments.

> **Supporting the holistic needs of children and families: key points**
>
> - Adults should act as a secure base and a safe haven for children. Insecure children may have difficulties with relationships, securely attached children usually develop good social and emotional skills
> - Insecurely attached children may sabotage developing relationships to protect themselves from rejection
> - When adults understand behaviour as communication, they can support the child by acting as a container for their feelings of vulnerability
> - When 'attention seeking' is reframed as 'attachment needing' behaviour it is seen as a symptom of internal conflict
> - Circles of Security is an approach built on attachment theory. The adult's role is to be emotionally strong, warm and available to intervene when appropriate, being "bigger and stronger, wiser and kind" (Marvin et al., 2002, p.110)
> - The key person role goes beyond a duty of care to an ethic of care. This includes fostering children's self-worth and identity
> - Worldwide studies by Rogoff have widened understanding of how children learn holistically in their unique culture. Taking a life world orientation approach will help you to appreciate these differences
> - Caregivers should bring their whole selves to working with children and families by drawing on the Head, Heart, Hands model
> - Applying Maslow's Hierarchy of Needs and Deci and Ryan's Self-Determination Theory can help meet children's psychological needs.

ADDITIONAL RESOURCES

- The Center on the Developing Child at Harvard University

This webpage has resources to support understanding of children's brain architecture, specifically the effects of trauma. It is not all theory, however, there are also practical ideas to try. Available at: https://developingchild.harvard.edu (Accessed 28 June 2024).

- Norman, A. (2023) *Using a person-centred approach in early years practice: a therapeutic guide for students.* London: Routledge

This book offers an alternative approach for those who work in an early year setting and want to take a holistic approach to practice and management.

- Plevin, R. (2017) *The fun teacher's tool kit: hundreds of ways to create a positive classroom environment & make learning FUN*. Needs Focussed Teaching. Life Raft Media Ltd

This book recognises that many children attending school are trauma experienced and although it offers practical ideas for making teaching fun, its purpose is to build relationships with children. There are free resources on the website too: https://www.needsfocusedteaching.com (Accessed 28 June 2024).

References

Ainsworth, M.D. and Bell, S.M. (1970) Attachment, exploration, and separation: illustrated by the behaviour of one-year-olds in a strange situation. *Child Development*, 41(1), pp. 49-67. doi: https://doi.org/10.2307/1127388.

Baron, S., Colomina, C., Pereira, T. and Stanley, T. (2019) *Strengths-based approach: practice framework and practice handbook*. Department of Health & Social Care, United Kingdom. Available at: https://assets.publishing.service.gov.uk/media/5c62ae87ed915d04446a5739/stengths-based-approach-practice-framework-and-handbook.pdf (Accessed 5 June 2024).

Bergin, C. and Bergin, D. (2009) Attachment in the classroom. *Educational Psychology Review*, 21(2), pp. 141-170. doi: 10.1007/s10648-009-9104-0.

Black, A.E. (2019) Treating insecure attachment in group therapy: attachment theory meets modern psychoanalytic technique. *International Journal of Group Psychotherapy*. doi: https://doi.org/10.1080/00207284.2019.1588073.

Bowlby, J. (1969) *Attachment and loss. Vol 1: Attachment*. New York. Basic Books.

Bowlby, J. (1973) *Attachment and loss. Vol. 2: Separation: anxiety and anger*. New York: Basic Books.

Bruce, T. (1987) *Early childhood education*. Oxford: Hodder Education.

Casement, P.J. (1985) *Learning from the patient*. London: The Guilford Press.

Cooper, P. (1999) *Understanding and supporting children with emotional and behavioural difficulties*. London: Jessica Kingsley Books.

Deci, E.L. and Ryan, R.M. (2000) The "what" and "why" of goal pursuits: human needs and the self-determination of behaviour. *Psychological Inquiry*, 11(4), pp. 227-268. doi: https://doi.org/10.1207/S15327965PLI1104_01.

Deci, E.L. and Ryan, R.M. (eds.) (2002) *Handbook of self-determination research*. New York: University of Rochester Press.

Department for Education (2023) *Early Years Foundation Stage Statutory Framework for Group and School-Based Providers*. Available at: https://assets.publishing.service.gov.uk/media/65aa5e42ed27ca001327b2c7/EYFS_statutory_framework_for_group_and_school_based_providers.pdf (Accessed 19 June 2024).

Elfer, P., Goldschmied, E. and Selleck, D. (eds.) (2003) *Key persons in the nursery*. London: David Fulton.

Foucault, M. (1977) *Discipline and punishment*. Translated by A. Sheridan. London: Penguin.

Frankl, V. E. (1959) *Man's search for meaning*. London: Hodder & Stoughton.

Geddes, H. (2017) Attachment behaviour and learning, in Colley, D. and Cooper, P. (eds.) *Attachment and emotional development in the classroom. Theory and practice*. London: Jessica Kingsley Books, pp. 37-48.

Goleman, D. (1996) *Emotional intelligence*. London: Bloomsbury.

Hancock, J. (2018) An emotional journey, in Gilbert, I. (ed.). *The working class. Poverty, education and alternative voices*. Carmarthen: Independent Thinking Press. pp. 81-90.

Harlow, H.F. and Zimmermann, R.R. (1958) The development of affective responsiveness in infant monkeys. *Proceedings of the American Philosophical Society*, 102, 501–509.

Hedegaard, M. (2009) Children's development from a cultural-historical approach: children's activity in everyday local settings as foundation for their development, *Mind, Culture, and Activity*, 16(1), pp. 64–81. doi: 10.1080/10749030802477374.

Hewitson, K. (2021) *If you can't reach them, you can't teach them. Building effective learning through relationships*. St Albans: Critical Publishing Ltd.

Huber, A., Hawkins, E. and Cooper, G. (2018) Circle of Security, in Lebow, J., Chambers, A. and Breunlin, D. (eds.) *Encyclopaedia of couple and family therapy*. New York: Springer, pp. 1–6. doi: 10.1007/978-3-319-15877-8_845-1.

Kaska, M. (2015). *Social pedagogy, an invitation*. London: Jacaranda Development.

Katz, L.G. and Chard, C. (2000) *Engaging children's minds: the project approach* 2nd edn. Stamford, CT: Ablex Publishing Corporation.

Kawamura, K.M. and Eisler, R. (2013) An interview with Nel Noddings, PhD. *Cross Cultural Management: An International Journal*, 20(2), pp. 1–10.

Lorenz, K. (1935) Der Kumpan in der Umwelt des Vogels. Der Artgenosse als auslösendes Moment sozialer Verhaltensweisen. *Journal für Ornithologie*, 83, pp. 137–215.

Marvin, R., Cooper, G., Hoffman, K. and Powell, B. (2002) The Circle of Security project: attachment-based intervention with caregiver-pre-school child dyads. *Attachment & Human Development*, 4(1), pp. 107–124. doi:10.1080/14616730252982491.

Maslow, A.H. (1943) A theory of human motivation. *Psychological Review*, 50(4), pp. 370–396.

Maxwell, A., McMahon, C., Huber, A., Reay, R.E., Hawkins, E. and Bryanne, B. (2021). Examining the effectiveness of Circle of Security Parenting (COS-P): a multi-site non-randomized study with waitlist control. *Journal of Child and Family Studies*, 30(5), pp. 1123–1140. doi: https://doi.org/10.1007/s10826-021-01932-4

Morris, K. (2015) *Promoting positive behaviour in the early years*. Maidenhead. Open University Press.

Munro, E. (2010) *The Munro Review of Child Protection Part One: a systems analysis*. Available at: https://assets.publishing.service.gov.uk/media/5a81e8a5e5274a2e8ab567a9/TheMunroReview-Part_one.pdf (Accessed 27 June 2024).

Naish, S., Oakley, A., O'Brien, H., Penna, S. and Thrower, D. (2023) *The A–Z of trauma-informed teaching*. London: Jessica Kingsley Publishers.

Noddings, N. (1995) Teaching themes of caring. *The Education Digest*, 61(3), p. 24.

Petrie, P., Boddy, J., Cameron, C., Heptinstall, E., McQuail, S., Simon, A. and Wigfall, V. (2008) *Pedagogy–a holistic, personal approach to work with children and young people, across services. Briefing Paper Update 2008*. London: Thomas Cranham Research Unit. Available at: https://www.thempra.org.uk/wp-content/uploads/2022/03/Petrie-et-al-Pedagogy-a-holistic-personal-approach-to-work-with-children.pdf (Accessed 25 June 2024).

Pietromonaco, P.R. and Powers, S.I. (2015) Attachment and health-related physiological stress processes. *Current Opinion in Psychology*, 1(1), pp. 34–39. doi: 10.1016/j.copsyc.2014.12.001.

Powell, B., Cooper, G., Hoffman, K. and Marvin, R. (2014) *The Circle of Security intervention: enhancing attachment in early parent-child relationships*. New York: Guilford.

Rogoff, B. (2003) *The cultural nature of human development*. Oxford: Oxford University Press.

Silber, K. (1965) *Pestalozzi: the man and his work*. London: Routledge & Kegan Paul.

Slade, R. (2019) Relationship sabotage in adults with low self-esteem from attachment trauma in childhood. *Family Perspectives*, 1(1), art. 11. Available at: https://scholarsarchive.byu.edu/familyperspectives/vol1/iss1/11 (Accessed 31May 24).

Stobbs, N. (2023) Social pedagogy as a lens for re-focussing ethics in education, in Solvason, C. and Elliott, G. (eds.) *Ethics in education*. Bradford: Ethics International Press Ltd, pp. 1–24.

The Circle of Security International (2022) *"Time In": a true-life example*. Available at: https://www.circleofsecurityinternational.com/2017/06/22/time-in-a-true-life-example (Accessed 18 June 2024).

Van Manen, M. (1991) *The tact of teaching*. London: The Althouse Press.

Wright, A. (2009). Every Child Matters: discourses of challenging behaviour, *Pastoral Care in Education*, 27(4), 279-290. doi: https://doi.org/10.1080/02643940903349344.

Part II
Exploring therapeutic approaches to supporting children and families

4
The importance of play

Introduction

It is a truth universally acknowledged that children benefit from play! In this chapter we discuss just how beneficial play can be in promoting cognitive and physical development as well as resilience and self-determined behaviour. We use the conceptual model of the learning zone to frame how play supports overall growth rather than a narrower focus on learning for academic success. We consider how play can support children to process trauma and how practitioners can adopt the attachment-based, therapeutic approach of PACE to support all children to feel valued and heard. We look at what this might look like in practice, with some practical tips that you can start implementing right away.

Biological, chemical and developmental benefits of play

Have you ever watched children move from one place to another? With a parent collecting dry cleaning, or a prescription from the chemist, perhaps. Utterly unself-consciously children will skip, spin, hopscotch, jump to avoid cracks in the pavement and generally bounce along; it's a joy to watch! From an energy expenditure perspective, however, bouncing is not nearly as efficient as walking, so what do children gain from it?

The additional steps taken when spinning strengthens children's bone density. It improves their physical health by increasing their heart rate and lung capacity without them noticing, storing up respiratory and cardio-vascular benefits in their bank of future adult healthiness (Kingston-Hughes, 2022).

As well as physical health, play also supports mental health. The drive to play develops in the limbic system of the brain, the part that controls what we need to survive, such as eating and reproduction, as well as our emotions and memories. When children are engrossed in play their brains release the natural chemicals, benzodiazepines, for example, Valium (Kingston-Hughes, 2022), the drug commonly prescribed for anxiety conditions. Depriving children of play potentially has the same impact on their wellbeing that depriving them of rest and food has on their physical development (Kingston-Hughes, 2022).

Play also supports cognitive development (Wood, 2013) both formally when used as a pedagogical approach (for example, playing hopscotch with children with the aim of teaching number recognition), and informally (for example, children could learn about volume and capacity when playing with water). Play with another person is the basis of social development. Babies seem pre-programmed to seek playful encounters; at just three weeks old they will respond by excitedly moving their arms and legs when greeting their caregiver. If the caregiver responds to these cues by smiling and mirroring a communicative dialogue ensues (Trevarthen, 2005) that builds attachment bonds and contributes to the foundations of a secure base (Ainsworth, 1969).

Risky play for growth

Risky play is defined as "thrilling and exciting forms of physical play that involve uncertainty and a risk of physical injury" (Sandseter, 2010, p.67). We all have our own boundary were fun meets scary, whether that's jumping across the gap between sofas, or riding a bike down a hill. Other aspects of risky play include playing with the natural elements (fire, wind, water and earth), rough and tumble play, play with tools and opportunities to "disappear" (Andrews, 2012, p.14).

Risky play and the learning zone

The Learning Zone Model (Thempra, n.d.), frequently used in social pedagogy, is a useful way of illustrating how freely chosen play can support children's resilience and wellbeing, particularly their risky play choices (see Figure 4.1).

In our comfort zone we feel safe in what is known; to grow, however, we must move into the learning zone. Once new experiences and learning have been accommodated by our brains, the comfort zone expands, leading to growth as we push a little further into the learning zone the next time we risk trying something new. Too much risk and we may tip into the panic zone, when the brain is flooded with anxiety, making learning and growth impossible.

Provided it is directed by the child risky play enables children to tentatively venture into the learning zone on their terms. Because they can retreat into the comfort zone at any point, they are never forced into the panic zone. A child may be comfortable exploring some woods with friends, for example. When encountering a tyre swing near a stream the child may sit in the tyre until they feel comfortable in interacting with a moving tyre. As the child moves

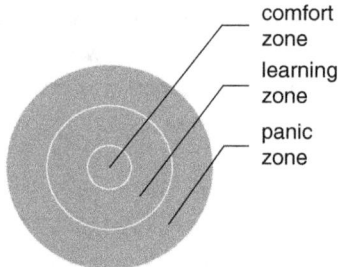

Figure 4.1 Simplified version of the Learning Zone Model (from Stobbs, 2019)

from the comfort zone to the learning zone, they may then stand on the tyre swing and ask another child to push them gently. As this sensation is accommodated further safe risks may be taken until the child is confident enough to swing over the stream. Joining in with like-minded friends who share the exhilaration has the bonus of being a bonding experience that enhances friendships and secure attachments.

Risky play and self-determined behaviour

When the degree of risky play is directed by the child fear of failure is minimal because they can retreat to the comfort zone when they want to, leading to feelings of *autonomy*. Children also access the play at a level that fits with their development, meaning that they can set their own personal challenges, enabling them to feel *competence*. When children play with peers and/or adults, feelings of belonging are evoked, satisfying the need for *relatedness*. Autonomy, competence and relatedness are the three basic psychological needs for self-determined behaviour as proposed by Deci and Ryan (2000), intrinsically motivating people to act intentionally according to their values and beliefs, even when this is not the easy option. This results in "higher quality behaviour and greater psychological wellbeing" (Deci & Ryan, 2000, p.243).

> **REFLECTIVE TASK**
>
> Have we become a risk averse society? Imagine watching a child use a plank of wood to bridge a small ditch about a metre high. How do you feel about them walking across their bridge?
> Now imagine the child repeatedly jumping on the plank bridge. If they continue there is a strong possibility that the plank will break, fall into the ditch along with the child. What is your reaction?
> Using the Three Ps, complete the table below to reflect on how risk averse you are.

Table 4.1 Levels of tolerance of risk using the three Ps

Question	Your response
Professional: Do I consider risk an important part of learning and wellbeing? What level of risk do I consider acceptable?	
Personal: What do I perceive as a risk? What are my reactions to perceived risk? How do I communicate these?	
Private: Where are my preferred boundaries when it comes to risk? Would I secretly rather children experienced no risk? What experiences have influenced my tolerance of risk?	

Play and resilience

There are many definitions of resilience but one that will resonate with those who work with children and families is that it is the "ordinary magic" (Masten, 2013) that comes from coping with everyday experiences. It is the ability to handle stress without becoming debilitated by it, or 'bouncing back' (Masten, 2013). Playing enables children to encounter failure in a safe way; through trial and error children learn that not giving up on something that you are personally invested in (for example, building a damn across a stream) comes together in the end as they learn from their mistakes. Angie Hart and Derek Blincow, with help from Helen Thomas, developed a resilience framework with five "potions" of magic to build resilience in children and young people, particularly those who face significant adversity (Hart & Aumann 2017, p.8). The five potions are: Basics, Belonging, Learning, Coping and Core Self, and play is a key ingredient in all of them. The resilience framework can be found at: https://resilience-pathway.co.uk/resilience-framework.

In the framework "Basics" is listed as "play and leisure", implicitly linking it to the right enshrined in article 31 of the UNCRC (United Nations Convention on the Rights of the Child) (UNICEF UK, 1989). The "good times and places" are referred to in "Belonging", summoning up happy memories and feelings of belonging children have when playing in places that are meaningful to them. Play is an implicit ingredient in the "Learning" potion, for example, when "making school life work as well as possible" for the young person; a key factor in effective pedagogy is taking a playful approach and allowing the child to test out any emergent learning for themself in play (Wood, 2013). Play is also an important ingredient in the "coping" potion, in particular "having a laugh" and "understanding boundaries and keeping within them", for example, in rough and tumble play children learn to wrestle happily without hurting the other person. In the final potion, "Core self", play is fundamental in "supporting the child to understand people's feelings", for instance, when role-playing a parent caring for a baby.

As has been outlined, everyday play has therapeutic benefits in and of itself since it promotes biological and cognitive growth, resilience and self-determined behaviour; "[it] … serve[s] to maintain health and wellbeing, in the sense of positive relationships, positive sense of self, connectedness and belonging" (Wood, 2008, p.117). Additionally, play can be used as a therapeutic intervention for children who have experienced trauma.

Play therapy

One way adults process difficult emotions is to talk them through with a trusted friend. For children who are still developing their emotional vocabulary this is an impossible task and more formal therapy delivered by play therapists may be beneficial. These professionals hold postgraduate qualifications accredited by the British Association of Play Therapists (BAPT) or Play Therapy UK (PTUK), often after completing a first degree in subjects such as Early Childhood Studies, Psychology or Psychiatric Nursing. Play therapists use methods such as art, drama, music, sensory activities, for example, playing with water, sand or clay, and imaginary play as a way for children to either to work through troubling experiences, often stored up in the sub-conscious (Senko & Bethany, 2019), in a safer, more detached way, or offer distraction from unavoidable difficulties. Approximately 20 per cent of children have some kind of mental, emotional or behavioural disorder (National Centre for Social Research, 2023) ranging from one-off incidents to extensive abuse, anxiety conditions, Attention Deficit Hyperactivity Disorder (ADHD), depression, grief and autism. Children who have accessed foster or adoption care services and those with a high incidence of adverse childhood experiences (ACEs) also frequently benefit from play therapy.

Health play therapists hold foundation degrees in a healthcare play specialism and mainly work in hospitals with children undergoing medical treatment, in the playroom or as part of other therapeutic play interventions.

Case study: health play specialist

Georgina Howden is a trained health play specialist and uses play to give children an outlet to work through their anxiety and stress. She now works in a special education mental health school where she uses daily play sessions to enhance wellbeing for the children. Here she writes about an experience with a child who needed ongoing hospital treatment.

> *Seven-year-old Alicia struggled with the regular blood tests necessary for managing her cystic fibrosis. I spent several weeks building a trusting relationship with Alicia and her mum on the ward, for example, making slime. This worked as an ice breaker, and I was able to slowly start talking with her about her blood tests. After some time spent playing and chatting, we agreed that she didn't want to be held still, she didn't like lots of people talking at once and she didn't want to see the blood at all. Each week I introduced something related to the blood test in a play activity --- for example, syringe painting, which was lots of messy fun. Once the painting was over, I showed Alicia how the 'butterfly' needle attaches to the syringe, and how only the tip of the needle draws out the blood, then we practised on a soft body doll.*
>
> *The following week I encouraged her to play with the 'numbing cream'. She put some on my hand and I put some on hers and we played a game. After 30 minutes we tested the cream with some 'scratchy' objects such as a toothbrush and a pencil. I asked, 'Can you feel this? The skin feels sleepy!' This was to help her to trust the topical anaesthetic.*
>
> *The next week we planned for her upcoming blood test. We made a poster with rules written by Alicia, for example, sitting on mum's lap - tummy to tummy, only two nurses in the room and a play specialist to play a distraction game with her on the iPad. During her blood test the phlebotomy team followed the plan. As the nurses did the blood test, she cried out but managed to stay still, which was a huge achievement. I reassured her that crying out can be a form of coping. When it was over, I took her to her to a cubicle to do some post procedure play. We made more slime! This helped with her recovery and soon she was feeling brighter.*
>
> *Alicia continued to build up her coping strategies at every appointment and over time the blood tests became easier for her.*

Critical questions

1. Before Georgina addressed Alicia's fear of needles what was her priority?
2. How did Georgina use therapeutic play techniques to de-mystify medical equipment?
3. How did Georgina help Alicia gain some control over her treatment? Why might feeling in control help when having a medical procedure?
4. Could these principles be applied more generally, for example, supporting children moving from a foster care setting to permanent adoption, or the transition to school from nursery? Are there any principles that do not apply?

Therapeutic play for practitioners

Some children need specialist intervention by qualified therapists, councillors or psychologists. These specialists are required to undergo clinical supervision to discuss their work, to relate theory to practice (education), to plan approaches, to be accountable for their practice and to reflect on any personal reactions aroused by their cases and ethical dilemmas (Play Therapy UK, n.d.). Children might need this more formal clinical intervention due to trauma caused by grief or abuse, resulting in anxiety, depression and even self-harm. It is beyond the scope of non-specialist therapeutic practitioners working with children to tackle these complexities and appropriate boundaries must be maintained; uninformed intervening can do further harm, however well meaning (see Chapter 1 for more on maintaining suitable boundaries).

Nonetheless, general therapeutic play approaches can be adapted for children's everyday care, benefitting those who need a little more support but fall below the threshold of clinical intervention. Although the brains of trauma-experienced children often revert to a 'fight or flight' response when put under stress (De Bellis & Zisk, 2014), the brain is malleable, and every positive interaction incrementally reconditions it to more measured responses.

PACE

PACE is a therapeutic approach underpinned by attachment theory (Ainsworth, 1969) developed by Dr Dan Hughes (Golding and Hughes, 2012) and was initially intended to be used with children who have experienced trauma, however, it is recognised by many practitioners as being consistent with their own values. It involves considering the whole child, taking into account everything that has happened or is happening to them and creating a safe environment that does not use shame as a basis for control. Patience is required but if used consistently PACE has potentially transformative effects on relationships between children and adults.

Each of the letters in the acronym stands for a different characteristic: Playfulness, Acceptance, Curiosity and Empathy.

Playfulness

Carr and Claxton (2002) define playfulness as being "joyful", a little "mischievous" and having a "glint in the eye" (p.15). To build a trusting relationship with the child you might collude to do an act of kindness for another member of the staff team you know such as making smiley faces on Post-its and surprising them by leaving them where they will be found and enjoyed. Adopting a playful attitude lightens the mood, defuses fear and inhibits the instinct to fight or flight because joy and fear cannot co-exist (Naish *et al.*, 2023). The child is more likely to share their feelings if the emotional temperature of the setting is relaxed and your manner is soft, using your eyes, eyebrows and mouth to demonstrate your interest in them. This means that if you need to remind the child about acceptable behaviour it does not crush them and trigger a fight or flight response. Instead, you model how to respond with proportionally and this encourages the child to do the same; being playful can make a directive less confrontational.

Acceptance

When a child has experienced trauma, they may test the boundaries of your regard for them to discover whether you accept them for who they are regardless of their actions (Walker, 2013). It is natural to seek a quick fix solution and apply a one size fits all technique that focuses on behaviour management rather than understanding the complexities of children's behaviour (Morris, 2015), but all children benefit from a considered and thoughtful response. This does not mean that unacceptable behaviour is tolerated, but the child needs to know that you accept their inner self, despite what their outer self is manifesting. Their inner self has been framed by stories they have been told about themselves, whether explicitly or internalised through experience and inference (Siegal, 2011). Children may use hurtful or emotionally raw words ('I'm useless', 'Nobody likes me', 'You hate me') and it is important not to correct or judge the child for their feelings. You may instead respond by saying, 'No wonder you're upset if you think nobody likes you. That must feel terrible. That might be why you kicked the chair over. Let's find another way to deal with those feelings.' Acceptance enables the relationship to continue despite any challenging behaviour (Winter, 2015).

Curiosity

Being genuinely curious about why a child has behaved as they have is not the same as demanding, '"What did you do that for!?' Rather, it is wondering aloud what may have triggered the behaviour. This means taking on a kind and speculative tone, making suggestions to the child, inviting them to take a step back and examine their actions as objectively as possible, as if you are working together to attribute the source. You could say, 'I wonder if you scribbled on Jackson's picture because you had a scribbly feeling inside, and it made your hands act all scribbly when you saw the picture Jackson had drawn of his mummy. What is that scribbly feeling like for you?'

Empathy

Goleman defines empathy as "the ability to know how another feels" (Goleman, 2005, p.96) and requires skilful interpretation of non-verbal cues such as facial expressions, tone of voice, gestures and posture. For practitioners this means being attuned to the emotions of the child and expressing this in small ways, such as mirroring their actions and reflecting their inner state, perhaps giving a high five when they are elated, or getting down to their level and gently wiping away their tears with a tissue when they are upset. In becoming attuned and showing empathy we should pause and consider what life must be like for that child, not only in the moment but from their whole experience of life. This is known in social pedagogy as "life-world orientation" and includes "a person's personality, strengths, likes, dislikes, their extended family and friends, culture, religion, place of upbringing and significant events in their life" (Kaska, 2015, p.43). Responding with empathy means considering the unique child; piecing together what you know and using that to understand the whole child, then imagining how you would feel if you were them. This might mean thinking what it would be like if you were a natural extravert but did not speak the dominant language and were unable to express yourself, for example. It goes beyond thinking how you would respond from your perspective of life (see Chapter 3 for more on life-world orientation).

Although you cannot change the circumstances of the child's lifeworld, by empathising with them you can act as a container for those circumstances (rather than offer reassurances that things will get better) and provide some comfort that they are not alone (Casement, 1985).

Critical questions

1. What mindset do you need to take when adopting a PACE approach?
2. How might you communicate your approach to parents without appearing critical of their practice?
3. Why is taking a whole team approach to PACE so important?
4. Why might taking a PACE approach be different from following a step-by-step process?

WINE sentence stems

A common approach used in conjunction with PACE is drawing on four potential sentence starters. Referred to as WINE sentence stems, they involve demonstrating your emotional availability by:

Wondering how the child is feeling, what they are thinking
Imagining what the child might be experiencing
Noticing their behaviour in a non-confrontational way
E showing **e**mpathy for how the child may be feeling.

These sentence prompts are appropriate when working with any child because they put relationships at the heart of each interaction and help us to connect with children before we correct them, inviting responsiveness rather than aggression (Siegal & Payne Bryson, 2016). The practice vignette below explores how playful approaches can be used in practice to support children who may be struggling.

Practice vignette

When I (Nicola) was a pre-school leader I used a playful approach to support and mentor a child struggling to form relationships with his peers. Below is a summary of what I did and the impact it had.

There were two four-year-old boys called Liam who attended pre-school, and I knew something had to be done when the children started to distinguish between them by calling one 'Naughty Liam'. I conducted and carefully analysed some observations of this Liam, noting that he spent most of his time in parallel play, interesting as typically four-year-olds would engage in social play by this stage.

Liam was obsessed with monsters and would spend long periods of time alone, highly tuned into a fantasy world populated by them. When other children came near him, he would roar or snap at them, pretending to be an imaginary creature. They either excluded or teased him, "there's a monster in the art cupboard!" as a way of getting an excited reaction from him, then would laughingly run away.

Liam's mother was very concerned and asked that all monster-related stories, games and small world toys be banned. She appeared relieved when leaving Liam at the beginning of the session but at collection time she struggled to make eye contact with him and seemed tense. Liam said his mother took his toys away when he would not share with his younger sister. The indications were that they had a strained relationship.

Liam's behaviour in pre-school was a puzzle. His highly active imagination did not enable him to connect with other children as would be expected. There had to be another reason why he so readily played alone in this way. Bloch (1978) suggests that children who develop an obsession with monsters are subconsciously afraid that their parents do not love them- one of the most terrifying fears a child can have. Transferring the fear onto monsters enables them to detach from their actual fear, preserving the parental love as complete and attainable.

Unable to influence Liam's relationship with his mother, I tried to improve Liam's relationship with his peers. We started twice weekly emotional coaching sessions focusing on one emotion per week (happiness, sadness, fear and anger) through playful scenarios, for example, examining photographs of children displaying various emotions, looking specifically at the facial features and body language. After identifying the emotions the children might be feeling we speculated about why they might feel this way and shared times when we had felt something similar.

We also used small world characters to recreate times when Liam had made poor social choices when interacting with his peers, such as getting into an argument if he disagreed with the rules. We practised new ways of responding, such as compromising or taking turns, how to join in the play without being irritating, and how to be resilient if the attempt to engage was unsuccessful. Throughout this time Liam grew more confident at identifying emotions, sharing with other children, and gradually stopped talking about monsters.

Liam then stopped being "Naughty Liam," and developed a supportive friendship. His mother seemed more relaxed when collecting him, particularly when she also developed a friendship with the mother of Liam's new friend.

Critical question

How did the playful approach support Liam to learn new behaviour without shaming him for his previous behaviour?

Implications for frontline practitioners

Children who have experienced trauma or neglect due to extreme poverty, conflict/war or abuse, for example, may not have enjoyed an attuned, playful relationship with a caregiver, or they may have been placated with technology. This can result in children presenting below the expected level of development for their age (Brown & Vaughan, 2010). They may also try to make others feel how they felt during their trauma, e.g., frightened, frozen out, isolated or helpless. Practising play skills with an understanding practitioner, however, can give children the opportunity to learn these relationship skills and build self-esteem and trust.

Everyday ideas for therapeutic play

The following suggestions are not intended to replace those of a qualified play therapist; they are instead good practice for supporting children to develop emotional resilience, process general anxieties and have sound wellbeing.

- Join their world. Children will learn to trust and bond with adults who can unselfconsciously hide behind a tree, spin under a wide sky, hold a telephone conversation using a banana, play chasing games or know the names of their favourite TV characters.
- If children play the same scenario repeatedly (for example, hiding from a 'baddie'), it is likely that this is their way of processing a fear or an actual event. You could guide them through different endings that give an element of control, for example, the police coming and taking the baddie away, or laughing at something the baddie does, for instance, tripping over a piece of rope.
- Play stop/go games such as 'What's the time, Mr. Wolf?' and 'Please, Mr. Crocodile ...". Use singing time to support self-regulation where children take turns at holding a double-sided card with green/go on one side and red/stop on the other.
- Bubble play. Running around popping bubbles is great for stress relief.
- Make an outline of a child's hand and draw a picture of someone who loves them or could help if they were in trouble on each finger.
- Make a stress ball by adding flour to a balloon, and then tying it with string/ribbon. Squeeze it when feeling anxious.
- Free-playing with playdough can be therapeutic in itself – having something to mould and squeeze with their hands is often relaxing. If a child opens up about something they are

afraid of (e.g., a monster under the bed) you can create the monster from playdough and then squash it flat with your hands, giving a sense of power and control.
- Sand play is a way of directing the trauma onto something other than the child. Using small world characters and other props (twigs, string, pebbles, shells, play vehicles, etc.) can enable children to re-create how they are feeling and start to process it.
- Create a worry box (for example, out of an old tissue box) with children. Ask them to write, draw or have you scribe any worries they have, then put them in the box. At agreed regular intervals review the list and give each worry a score between 1 and 10 where 1 is low and 10 is severe. See whether the list moves over time. 'Containing' worries like this enables the child to carry on with their lives without being overwhelmed by anxious thoughts.

Conclusion

Play supports the development of children's academic skills, resilience and self-determined behaviour. Play can also be used in a therapeutic way to support children process trauma, adversity and grief. Non-specialist therapeutic practitioners who value supporting the whole child may choose to adopt the playful, attachment-based approach PACE and use WINE statements to foster meaningful relationships built on trust and acceptance. Practitioners have a crucial role in working with trauma-experienced children and play is one of the simplest and cheapest ways of helping children re-gain their equilibrium and sparkle.

The importance of play: key points

- There are biological, chemical and developmental benefits to play that support children's physical, mental and cognitive development.
- Risky play can foster growth and provide opportunities to act in a self-determined way by meeting the three psychological needs of autonomy, competence and relatedness.
- Play enables children to encounter failure in a safe way and can support the development of resilience.
- Play therapy delivered by qualified play therapists may be beneficial for children who need professional help to process traumatic experiences.
- PACE is a holistic, play-based approach that can be adopted by all practitioners to support children navigate general anxiety and fear.
- Emotional coaching through playful encounters can successfully promote understanding of how to foster meaningful relationships.
- Empathetic non-specialist therapeutic practitioners can use play activities with therapeutic aspects to help children feel a sense of belonging and trust and develop emotional resilience.

> **ADDITIONAL RESOURCES**
>
> - Engen, M., Søberg Bjerre, L. and Jensen, M. (2020). Play therapy insights into everyday social pedagogical practice in residential childcare, *International Journal of Social Pedagogy*, 9(1), pp.1–14. doi: https://doi.org/10.14324/111.444.ijsp.2020.v9.x.014
>
> This article considers the benefits of play therapists and social pedagogues working together to support trauma-experienced children in residential care.
>
> - Fearn, M. (2021) Accessing the therapeutic powers of play: a guide for playworkers. Play Wales. Available from: https://www.traumainformedschools.co.uk/images/Accessing_the_therapeutic_powers_of_play.pdf (Accessed 19 March 2024).
>
> A seven-page information sheet summarising how play can be used to support children experiencing anxiety.
>
> - Lowenstein, L. (2011) *Favourite therapeutic activities for children, adolescents and families: practitioners share their most effective interventions*. Toronto: Champion Press. Available at: https://proceduresonline.com/trixcms1/media/8424/favourite-therapeutic-activities-for-children.pdf (Accessed 19 March 2023).
>
> The book details many play interventions to spark ideas for practice.
>
> - Naish, A., Oakley, A., O'Brien, H., Penna, S. and Thrower, D. (2023) *The A-Z of trauma-informed teaching. strategies and solutions to help with behaviour and support for children aged 3-11*. London: Jessica Kingsley Publishers.
>
> A dip-in toolkit for what trauma-informed teaching looks like and a comprehensive compilation of behaviours you may come across.

References

Ainsworth, M.D. (1969) Object relations, dependency, and attachment: a theoretical review of the infant-mother relationship. *Child Development*, 40(4), pp. 969–1025. doi: https://doi.org/10.2307/1127008.

Andrews, M. (2012) *Exploring play for early childhood studies*. London: Sage.

Bloch, D. (1979) *"So the witch won't eat me?" Fantasy and the child's fear of infanticide*. London: Burnett Books in association with Andre Deutch.

Booth-LaForce, C. and Oxford, M.L. (2008) Trajectories of social withdrawal from Grades 1 to 6. Prediction from early parenting, attachment and temperament. *Developmental Psychology*, 44(5), pp.1298–1313.

Brown, S. and Vaughan, C. (2010) *Play, how it shapes the brain, opens the imagination and invigorates the soul*. London: Penguin/Random House.

Carr, M. and Claxton, G. (2002) Tracking the development of learning dispositions, *Assessment in Education: Principles, Policy and Practice*, 9(1), pp. 9–37.

Casement, P.J. (1985) *Learning from the patient*. London: The Guilford Press.

De Bellis, M.D., and Zisk A. (2014) The biological effects of childhood trauma. *Child and Adolescent Psychiatric Clinics of North America*, 23(2), pp.185–222. doi:https://doi.org/10.1016/j.chc.2014.01.002.

Deci, E. L. and Ryan, R.M. (2000) The 'What' and 'Why' of goal pursuits: human needs and the self determination of behavior, *Psychological Inquiry*, 11(4), pp. 227–268. doi: 10.1207/S15327965PLI1104_01.

Early Education (2021) *Birth to five matters: non-statutory guidance for the Early Years Foundation Stage*. Available at: https://birthto5matters.org.uk (Accessed 27 February 2024).

Golding, K.S. and Hughes, D.A. (2012) *Creating loving attachments: parenting with PACE to nurture confidence and security in the troubled child*. London: Jessica Kingsley Publishers.

Goleman, D. (2005) *Emotional intelligence*. 10th edn. New York: Bantam Books.

Hart, A. and Aumann, K. (2017) Briefing paper: *Building child and family resilience – Boingboing's resilience approach in action*. Totnes: Research in Practice. Available at: https://www.boingboing.org.uk/wp-content/uploads/2019/04/Building-child-and-family-resilience.pdf (Accessed 7 September 2023).

Kaska, M. (2015) *Social pedagogy, an invitation*. London: Jacaranda Recruitment Ltd.

Kingston-Hughes, B. (2022) *A very unusual journey into play*. London: Sage.

Masten, A.S. (2013) *Ordinary magic: resilience in development*. London: The Guilford Press.

Morris, K. (2015) *Promoting positive behaviour in the early years*. Maidenhead: Open University Press.

National Centre for Social Research, (2023) *Children and young people's mental health in 2023*. Available at: https://natcen.ac.uk/publications/children-and-young-peoples-mental-health-2023?gad_source=1&gclid=CjwKCAjw_LOwBhBFEiwAmSEQAV6gip5yVO2uXTIBAqVzK1CARHQ2hBOXKxRyMutoN2zpNq4yTwrTBBoCdTUQAvD_BwE (Accessed 3 April 2024).

Oden, S. and Asher, S.R. (1977) Coaching children in social skills for friendship making. *Child Development*, 48, 495–506.

Play Therapy UK (n.d.) *Clinical supervision*. Available at: https://playtherapy.org.uk/clinical-supervision (Accessed 4 October 2023).

Sandseter, E.B.H. (2010) It tickles my tummy! Understanding children's risk taking in play through reversal theory, *Journal of Early Childhood Research*, 8(1), pp. 67–88. doi: 10.1177/1476718X09345393.

Senko K, Bethany H. (2019) PLAY THERAPY: an illustrative case. *Innovations in Clinical Neuroscience*, 16(5-6), pp. 38–40.

Siegal, D. (2011) *Mindsight: transform your brain with the new science of kindness*. London: One World Publications.

Siegal, D. and Payne Bryson, T. (2016) *No-drama discipline: the whole brain way to calm the chaos and nurture your child's developing mind*. New York: Bantam Books.

Stobbs, N. (2019) The play, pedagogy, learning and teaching divide: can we close the gap? *TACTYC Reflections Papers*. Available at: https://tactyc.org.uk/reflections (Accessed 4 October 2023).

Thempra (n.d.) The learning zone model, key concepts in social pedagogy practice. Available at: https://www.thempra.org.uk/social-pedagogy/key-concepts-in-social-pedagogy/the-learning-zone-model (Accessed 4 October 2023).

Trevarthen, C. (2005). First things first: infants make good use of the sympathetic rhythm of imitation, without reason or language. *Journal of Child Psychotherapy*, 31(1), pp. 91–113. doi:https://doi.org/10.1080/00754170500079651.

UNICEF UK (1989) *The United Nations Convention on the Rights of the Child*. Available at: https://downloads.unicef.org.uk/wp-content/uploads/2010/05/UNCRC_PRESS200910web.pdf?_ga=2.78590034.795419542.1582474737-1972578648.1582474737 (Accessed 7 September 2023).

Walker, P. (2013) *Complex PTSD: from surviving to thriving: a guide and map for recovering from childhood trauma*. Scotts Valley, CA: CreateSpace Independent Publishing Platform.

Winter, K. (2015) Supporting positive relationships for children and young people who have experience of care. *Insights*, 20 February. Available at: https://www.iriss.org.uk/resources/insights/supporting-positive-relationships-children-young-people-experience-care (Accessed 13 February 2024).

Wood, E. (2008) Everyday play activities as therapeutic and pedagogical encounters, *European Journal of Psychotherapy and Counselling*, 10(2), pp. 111–120. doi: 10.1080/13642530802076151.

Wood, E. (2013) *Play, learning and the early childhood curriculum*. London: Sage.

5
The role of creativity in supporting those who have experienced adversity

Introduction

Despite all the clips of cute cats and dogs on social media, have you ever seen them compose a piece of music, or paint a beautiful sunset? Being creative is uniquely human and involves more than instinctive behaviour. Just looking around as I sit at my desk, I see my phone, a ball-point pen and my glasses case; all these were imagined and then created by designers and developers. Creativity is essential for continued advancement. But creativity has another potential super-power; it can bridge the gap between anger, trauma, adversity and grief to healing, resolution and restoration. In this chapter, we explore some ways this happens, what our role might be and what we should avoid.

Definition of creativity

'I'm not creative' is a common response when talking about creativity, perhaps because it is associated with 'the arts', music, drama, art, dance, literature, etc., although it is also essential for advances in science, maths, politics and technology, all areas of life in fact (National Advisory Committee on Creative and Cultural Education (NACCCE) 1999, p.29).

There are many definitions of creativity, but the one given by NACCCE accommodates these wide-ranging aspects: "Imaginative activity fashioned so as to produce outcomes that are both original and of value" (NACCE, 1999, p.30).

When analysed, creativity comprises four characteristics (as seen in Figure 5.1):

1. **Imaginative:** being innovative, e.g., by combining ideas in unexpected ways or in new areas
2. **Purposeful:** applying imagination to meet a goal or create an outcome
3. **Original:** either individual (compared to what the person has created previously), relatively original (compared to others) or historically, (compared to what happened in the past)
4. **Valuable:** be of worth, e.g., useful, effective, fulfilling or enjoyable.

(Hasley et al., 2006)

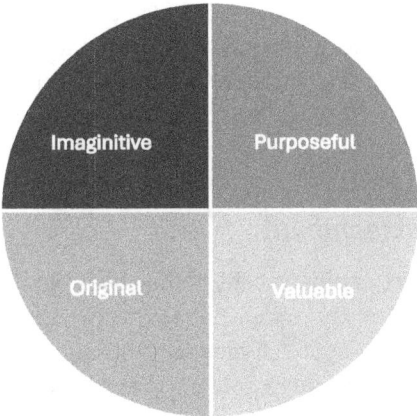

Figure 5.1 Four characteristics of creativity

Developmental benefits of creativity

The Cultural Learning Alliance (2017) reviewed research to determine any benefits for children engaging in the arts, publishing their "compelling and comprehensive" findings:

1. Participation in structured arts activities can increase cognitive abilities by 17%.
2. Learning through arts and culture can improve attainment in Maths and English.
3. Learning through arts and culture develops skills and behaviour that lead children to do better in school.
4. Students from low-income families who take part in arts activities at school are three times more likely to get a degree.
5. Employability of students who study arts subjects is higher and they are more likely to stay in employment.
6. Students from low-income families who engage in the arts at school are twice as likely to volunteer.
7. Students from low-income families who engage in the arts at school are 20% more likely to vote as young adults.
8. Young offenders who take part in arts activities are 18% less likely to re-offend.
9. Children who take part in arts activities in the home during their early years are ahead in reading and Maths at age nine.
10. People who take part in the arts are 38% more likely to report good health.

(Cultural Learning Alliance, 2017, p.2)

If engaging in the arts produces these results there is reason enough to value them, however, the benefits extend far beyond these instrumental outcomes.

Creativity and processing trauma

Do you ever wish you could 'gift' children self-esteem, good mental health, wellbeing and relationships? Or that we could just tell them to feel better, be better, change their behaviour or emotions and it would effortlessly happen? Sadly, this is rarely the case (Camic, 2008). What we can do, however, is create conditions for children to process traumatic experiences enabling them to move forward and improve their overall wellbeing. Creative activities can be a medium for this (Parker, 2020), for example, in building bonds of attachment in early childhood.

Creativity and early attachment

Depression and anxiety affect parents' ability to bond with their child, (Davies et al., 2021), therefore early intervention is key to circumventing the longer-term dangers associated with an insecure attachment, such as poor self-identity, self-regulation and social and emotional skills (Belsky & Fearon, 2002). Thankfully, poor early attachment is not irreversible (Belsky & Fearon, 2002), and art therapy has been shown to be effective in improving the relationship between parents and children (Bruce & Hackett, 2021).

During the COVID-19 pandemic there were few opportunities to participate in art therapy sessions due to social distancing restrictions, meaning that some parents already at risk of depression and anxiety were at further risk due to isolation (Wu et al., 2020). A research team at the University of Dundee was concerned that the vulnerable families (mainly single mothers and babies) they were working with would no longer have access to in-person art therapy so decided to deliver art boxes with resources and suggested activities to the families' homes (Armstrong & Ross, 2022).

At the end of the project all parents reported increased positive mental health and wellbeing, and being more playful with their children, a known factor in improving attachment bonds (Bigelow et al., 2010). Several parents reported that exploring the art activities with their children made them feel that they were being a good parent, as well as distracting them from worries, and all stated that their babies seemed happier and more confident (Armstrong & Ross, 2022). Parents recalled babies' excitement when the art boxes were brought out, suggesting anticipation of a good experience. Parents also noticed that their babies grew in agency when choosing art materials. Significantly, the fact that the parents picked up on these new behaviours suggests that they had started to view the babies as distinct individuals that they could connect with (Stern, 1985) and were able to "mentalise" about their mental state and intentions, all things associated with stronger attachments (Meins et al., 2001). In addition, the parents shared photographs of the art produced with family, indicating that they felt successful in their parenting abilities, itself suggesting self-satisfaction and wellbeing.

This demonstrates that sharing even simple art activities can increase attachment bonds between parents and babies and improve mental health and wellbeing.

Music and belonging

If you have ever been to a concert where everyone sang along to well-loved songs, you will know that music has the power to lift our spirits, move us to tears and make us feel part of something bigger than ourselves (Bang, 2016). It feels good because of the release of the mood enhancing chemical dopamine, triggered when we feel the connection to music (Zaatar et al., 2023). When this happens on a large scale, the effects can be powerful.

The Loud and Clear project, which consisted of looked-after children and their carers/adoptive parents hoped to tap into some of this potential power (Humphrey, 2020). The facilitators took a social pedagogy approach, where educational, relationship and care needs are considered as a whole (Chambers & Petrie, 2009). The children and their carers/adoptive parents explored musical instruments together, as well as socialising and connecting with others in similar situations, which fostered a sense of belonging and guarded against isolation, a contributor to poor mental health (Christiansen et al., 2021). During the sessions children and carers/adoptive parents engaged in bonding activities such as tickling, cuddling and dancing together (Humphrey, 2020).

At the end of the project some parents continued the musical activities at home; however, there were many other benefits beyond increased musicality. The activities had helped to build attachments and establish routines, for example, singing the group 'tidy-up' song when it was time to tidy away at home. Lullabies were sung at bedtime and provided a shared meaning, so important in the early stages of adoption (Humphrey, 2020). Other projects using group music activities with children at risk found it fostered a sense of purpose and increased confidence and self-esteem (Wood et al., 2013).

Meeting the three psychological needs through creativity

As discussed in Chapter 3, self-determination theory (Deci & Ryan, 2000) maintains there are three basic psychological needs, autonomy, relatedness and competence. A psychological need is more than just really wanting something (for example, a designer handbag or a new bike). These basic needs are defined as a "psychological nutrient that is essential for individuals' adjustment, integrity, and growth" (Vansteenkiste et al., 2020, p.1). If our need for autonomy, relatedness and competence is not met we become passive and/or defensive (Ryan & Deci, 2000). This theory can be applied to humans across the life span regardless of culture or personality (Vansteenkiste et al., 2020).

Creative activities have the potential to facilitate these three basic psychological needs. In the music and art activities discussed, the environment promoted *relatedness*, both within families and the wider community. Additionally, there is evidence of *competence*, both in terms of artistic and musical skill and as a new parent, for example. Although guided by facilitators there were opportunities for children and parents to use their *autonomy*, both in the group deciding to participate, and at home when they chose to apply what they had experienced to their own context.

Flow

Being creative can potentially induce a state of flow. Csikszentmihalyi pioneered the development of the flow theory and, like the self-determination theory (Ryan & Deci, 2000), it is applicable to people of all ages, cultures and personalities (Csikszentmihalyi,1990). Characteristics of flow include:

- Challenge-skill balance: Perceived equivalence of the activity's demands and the skills one possesses
- Clear goals: Knowing what to do in the activity
- Unambiguous feedback: Availability of instant feedback about performance

- Automaticity: Sense of performing automatically, instinctively
- Concentration: Narrowly focusing on the task/activity
- Sense of control: Feeling in control of performance
- Loss of self-consciousness: The absence of concerning self-evaluation
- Transformation of time: Passing of time seeming different
- Autotelic experience: Finding the experience intrinsically rewarding; enjoyable.

(cited in Parsons *et al.*, 2023, p.138)

When in a state of flow, we are totally involved and forget about the world beyond our activity, this gaining respite from our troubles. Whether people engage in creative activities individually or as a group, their absorbing nature improves mood and increases motivation and overall life satisfaction (Parsons *et al.*, 2023).

Critical questions

- Are there any activities that you do where you feel a sense of flow?
- How do you feel after doing these activities?
- Do you feel a sense of flow when you are on your own, or with others?
- Engaging with screens can momentarily distract from worries; how does this relate to flow activities?
- How can you increase your moments of flow?

The practice vignette below shows how creativity can be used to support children's emotional wellbeing.

Practice vignette

Natasha is an emotional literacy support assistant (ELSA) in a school nurture unit, working with Riley, whose mother was only 16 years old when she gave birth to him. Riley has lived with his grandparents for the past seven years, but his mother is in a new relationship and wants Riley to move in with her and her new partner. Riley's behaviour has become disruptive, and he frequently uses bad language, stands on furniture or walks out of class.

When Riley first came to the nurture unit, he picked up paper and pens and drew a house with four square windows, a triangle roof and smoke coming from the chimney, but no door. Natasha decided to implement a therapeutic intervention called "Drawing and Talking" (see Tait and Reilly (2021) for a report on this therapeutic intervention), a safe way to explore and communicate feelings in a non-confrontational way.

Natasha sees Riley once a week for 12 weeks. At first, he looks down all the time and does not smile. His drawings are of explosions and bombs, monsters and storms. Over time he starts to talk about his images, although there is no logical narrative to them. In their fifth session Riley begins to depict his grandparents, mother and new stepfather crying and himself as a superhero with tornadoes for legs. As he draws, he speaks about leaving his grandparents "all alone" and his mixed feelings about having a "normal" mum and dad paired with the worry that they will not get along well together.

Over the next three sessions Riley's drawings include two houses with windows, chimneys and doors and Natasha recognises that Riley is beginning to imagine being welcome in both his grandparents' and his mum's house. He begins to draw frames around his pictures, sunshine and bridges between the two houses. His grandparents, mum and stepfather are smiling, and Riley also draws a dog, adding that he hopes he can have a puppy when he moves to his new home.

Natasha can see that Riley feels in control of his emotions as he anticipates the move in a more positive light. His behaviour is far more settled, he has started to make friends with other children and is much calmer overall.

Critical question

What role did Drawing and Talking play in enabling Riley to process his conflicting emotions?

Resilience and drama

A characteristic of resilient people is that they can name and analyse their own and others' emotions (Pawlicka & Kaźmierczak, 2018, p.17). They use positive emotions when circumstances are against them (Tugade & Fredrickson, 2004), such as re-framing negative experiences as learning opportunities. Resilient children are open to experiences, even when they are new or potentially frightening (Ogińska-Bulik & Kobylarczyk, 2015), and so everyday setbacks are less likely to get them down (Russell, 2018).

Resilient people also have an internal locus of control, i.e., they believe they can affect their own circumstances. The opposite is an external locus of control, a belief that the power to change their situation lies with others or their environment, that they are unlucky or that this is their fate (Rotter, 1966). Resilient people are motivated to improve their situation, leading to a positive outlook on life (Kobylarczyk & Ogińska-Bulik, 2015). Children with an internal locus of control generally show more resilience after experiencing a traumatic event compared to those with an external locus of control (Kobylarczyk & Ogińska-Bulik, 2015).

Role play can temporarily impose an internal locus of control on children, releasing them from emotional baggage and enabling them to experience confidence and control. Conversely, those with high self-esteem may develop a new understanding and empathy for others when portraying a character who lacks confidence (Russell, 2018) resulting in less impulsivity or judging others harshly (Folostinaa et al., 2015).

Role play enables children to explore unprocessed issues that may impact on a fictional character's behaviour. Because action alternates between emotional engagement and a "rational distancing" it facilitates a "re-examining of what is viewed as failures or misfortunes and any other stereotypical assumptions" (Russell, 2018, p.109). In other words, you can be in character depicting different emotions one minute, but then come out of character and objectively explore the character's motivation and reasons for their emotions, thus contributing to new insights and learning.

Drama encourages risk-taking, building trust with others and becoming part of something meaningful, all known to support wellbeing (Christiansen et al., 2021). Performing for others requires controlling nerves and becoming comfortable with anxiety (Sawyer, 2015), which is more manageable if everyone around you is also nervous. Feeling anxious on your own is isolating, but having butterflies in your tummy along with everyone else is almost exciting!

Art as therapy

Children who have experienced significant trauma need clinical treatment by qualified professionals to prevent the development of Post Traumatic Stress Disorder (PTSD) (Gillies et al., 2013). Mildly traumatic experiences, however, such as the death of a pet, a humiliating experience or a non-life-threatening injury, can be processed through engaging in artistic activities that provide a vehicle for safe self-expression when talking is difficult (Gordon, 2007). Over time this helps children "absorb" the trauma, adjust and move forward (Mutch & Latai, 2019, p.232). By focusing energy on what is being created, dark thoughts can be explored in a non-triggering way and the cycle of re-living the trauma interrupted (Orr, 2007), allowing change and growth (Parker, 2020).

Avenues of hope

Drawing on Lee's four stages of psychosocial transition from trauma (Lee, 1970, cited in Appleton, 2001, p.8) Valerie Appleton devised the Avenues of Hope approach (Appleton, 2001) when working with children who had sustained burn injuries. It asserts that as part of the journey to resolution children typically transition through four stages: impact, retreat, acknowledgement and reconstruction (Appleton, 2001, p.7). Appleton added a goal for each stage-1. creating continuity, 2. building alliances, 3. overcoming anxiety and 4. fostering meaning.

This approach is useful for practitioners planning for children who have experienced mild trauma.

Table 5.1 A conceptual model of the four stages of psychosocial transition from trauma incorporated into art therapy, based on Appleton's Avenues of Hope (2001)

Stage	Child's behaviour	Your role/strategy
Stage 1: impact. *Goal:* creating continuity	Shock Heightened fear, anxiety, sorrow Disassociation from reality	Comfort and reassure Return to regular routines, e.g., mealtimes, bedtimes, returning to school Distraction from traumatic memories. Look for positives, e.g., the event is over, or there is respite from it Find a safe way to begin to process the event, associated emotions and aftermath

(Continued)

Table 5.1 (Conitnued)

Stage	Child's behaviour	Your role/strategy
Stage 2: retreat *Goal:* building alliances	Out of character behaviour, e.g., bedwetting (or day wetting), withdrawal, listlessness, hyperactivity, impulsivity or anger	Regard behaviour as a reaction to unprocessed trauma rather than 'naughty' Use relaxation techniques to prepare children for art sessions Engage in art activities Conclude with opportunities for others, e.g., parents, to listen to and view their child's work, facilitating community bonds
Stage 3: acknowledgement *Goal:* overcoming anxiety	Children start to manage their fears. They can regulate emotions, reframe the event in a more positive light and problem solve Pragmatic conversations, e.g., about the practicalities of their artistic creations (colours, etc.) A sense of distance from the event starts to develop	Work alongside the children and engage in their conversations
Stage 4: reconstruction *Goal:* fostering meaning	Sense of closure – the traumatic event becomes part of their past	Display the artwork if that is the children's wish. Some may want to symbolically burn, bury or throw away their work

Creating a safe space; guidelines for success

Creating a safe and nurturing space is a key aspect of the journey from trauma to healing (Mutch & Latai, 2019) and needs careful consideration. Here are some guidelines for success:

- Stress that all activities are optional, and children can opt out anytime (Mutch & Latai, 2019)
- Rather than go straight to paper-based activities explore difficult topics indirectly first, using stories, drama or dance to warm up and stimulate ideas (Mutch & Latai, 2019)
- For children unaccustomed to exercising autonomy consider doing a low-stakes, joint activity, possibly with a key person. Something requiring no instructions, such as engaging in a 'mindful' colouring book, can be effective in breaking the ice (Parker, 2000)
- Emphasise that there is no right or wrong response (MacDonald *et al.*, 2023). Be attuned to each child's confidence regarding their artistic abilities and adjust support accordingly. (Craft *et al.*, 2001)
- Meet in a neutral space not associated with painful memories (MacDonald *et al.*, 2023)
- Be sensitive to the cultural context. Western, neo-liberal cultures value independence and individuality; co-construction and collaboration, common in in Far Eastern cultures, may be appropriate for larger scale projects but some families may see this as inferior to individual work (Craft *et al.*, 2001).

The most important factor when using creative activities in therapeutic ways, however, is the development of genuine relationships with the children and families (Parker, 2020).

Building authentic relationships

Due to the difficulties insecurely attached children have with forming trusting relationships (Pietromonaco & Powers, 2015), they could feel anxious about attending creative therapeutic sessions. The same may also be true for the practitioners (Parker, 2020).

The social pedagogy concept of the three Ps is a useful framework for establishing appropriate warm relationships between practitioners, children and families. The model consists of three spheres: *professional*, *personal* and *private* (Jappe, 2010, cited in Kaska, 2015). Our *professional* self refers to our professional knowledge, for example, the best theory to apply, official processes or policies, research and experience. The *personal* relates to the 'human' side of our personality, for example, our likes and dislikes, challenges and experiences or humour. This might involve sharing our anxieties, for example, "I don't know why, but I always feel a bit nervous when meeting people I don't know". Letting your guard down can make you feel a little exposed, but it can be a good way to begin relationship building (Parker, 2020).

The *private* sphere concerns aspects of ourselves that would not be helpful for the child or young person to know, such as our own traumas, personal beliefs or mistakes. These should only be shared with those we are close to.

The Common Third

In social pedagogy consciously engaging in new activities and environments with others enables relationships to be strengthened and new skills to be learned. This is known as "The Common Third" (Kaska, 2015, p.52). When the focus is on the joint activity the traditional teacher/pupil relationship, with its inherent power hierarchies, is disrupted, and personal connections of trust develop naturally.

When things go wrong

Sometimes no matter what support we offer a child to help them through stress or trauma nothing seems to work. In this situation we should remain constant – the child may be testing you to ascertain whether they are accepted unconditionally (Parker, 2020). After a difficult session check with a parent or key person about what might be going on in the child's life, for example, an upcoming medical appointment, family worries or a broken sleep pattern. Be prepared to involve another person who has a good relationship with the child in the sessions; their encouragement and light-hearted banter could ease the atmosphere. Teamwork and reflective practice are key when working with children and discussing with others why some strategies were effective on some occasions but not others can be very helpful Parker, 2020).

Responding to children's sadness

A common side-effect of working with trauma-experienced children is that we absorb their sadness and despair (Parker, 2020) (see Chapter 11 for more on this). It may be tempting to try to minimise the child's pain in an attempt to cheer them up. As mentioned in Chapter 3, however, children need adults who will act as 'containers' for their difficult emotions rather than dismiss them (Casement, 1985). Robbins (2001, cited in Parker, 2020, p.11), stresses "growth occurs from the process of going through the pain of an unmet stage of development . . . to rob a patient of his [sic] anger, pain, and despair, no matter how well intentioned, is to do a disservice". Trauma is our body's response when our nervous system cannot process something quickly enough (Sellers, 2020). Children must be allowed to process the traumatic experience at a pace that the nervous system can cope with.

During this process children will display upsetting emotions, and it is particularly important to bring the session to a safe conclusion. Perhaps ask the child to summarise what they have felt or, if necessary, do this for them. The child needs to know that you can bear their pain and not shrink away, that you hear and understand them (Parker, 2020). Over time children's confidence in themselves and in you will increase, enabling them to take control of their narrative, moving through their grief and loss. As they cast off the 'passive victim' role sometimes imposed by adults, they will see themselves as 'survivors' rather than 'victims' and begin to heal (Gibbs *et al.*, 2013).

Case study: person-centred therapist

Carla Rettalick is a trained person-centred therapist. Having gone through a difficult journey of her own she is now passionate about helping others who want healing and comfort during tough times. Here Carla shares how she supported nine-year-old Max who was struggling with a major life event.

> Max came for counselling following the breakup of his parents' marriage. Max's mother, Theresa, had instigated the split when her husband physically abused her and Max's older brother. Max's father lived nearby and although Max still saw his father frequently, he felt very angry about the situation – he loved his mother, father and brother and felt conflicted loyalties.
>
> In our first session Max entered the room and was immediately drawn to playing with a Rubix cube. This became the pattern for future sessions, Max talking about what was on his mind while his hands were busy with the Rubix cube, taking pressure off having to make eye contact.
>
> During one session Max mentioned that he liked music, so the next time he came I brought out some pencils that were also drumsticks. I played some music on my phone, and he drummed along while talking to me. Max enjoyed this a lot, and we did this for a few consecutive sessions. One day, Max said that the music reminded him of his dad. I decided to use the 'anger iceberg', a tool that helps therapists and clients dig down into what other feelings might be hidden beneath the anger. This was very helpful, and Max circled several words on the anger iceberg worksheet. During the next few weeks, we explored those feelings. As the anger came out, Max wrote the hidden emotions he had identified on pieces of paper, then scrunched them up and threw them in the bin. This reduced him to tears, a barrier that he had not previously let down. He would say out loud, "I am nervous" and then throw the emotion in the bin, and if he missed the target he would try again, literally binning his emotions.

After that session, Max was different. He came in smiling and no longer wanted the Rubix cube. He said he had started a new hobby, origami, so over the next few months we made origami sculptures together, sometimes him teaching me and sometimes the other way around. There was a shift in our relationship; he used to be the client and me the knowledgeable therapist, but it became genuinely equal. Max loved the responsibility of finding new things for us to create and we built big fort constructions all over the floor as we spoke about his losses. Later, he started to talk about the future and of perhaps becoming an engineer.

Just as Max was gaining some equilibrium, he suffered another setback when Theresa decided to emigrate to Australia. He was crushed by this news and again felt conflicted about missing his father and wanting to be near his mother's extended family. Devasted by considering everything he would lose, Max returned to the comfort of the Rubix cube. He made no eye contact and everything he spoke about was negative. Max's father refused to give the boys' passports to Theresa, resulting in a court case.

Theresa was in tears as she collected Max one day, upset that he had regressed after doing so well. I asked her if she had ever spoken to her ex-husband rather than communicating through a solicitor. She replied that she had not and immediately sent him a message asking if he would meet her for lunch. He agreed and Theresa explained her reasons for wanting to emigrate; the following day Max's father returned the passports.

Max was so happy that everything was resolved. In our second to last session, I knew he was healed when he asked, "Carla, how are you?" It was no longer all about him; when people are in their zone of despair, they don't even notice you.

Max did emigrate and sent me a Zoom invitation to attend his Bar Mitzvah, which was very special to watch.

Critical Questions

- How did Carla work with Max's creativity to support his emotional processing?
- Carla talks of "equality" within the therapeutic relationship. How does creativity support this dynamic?
- How can you use creativity to support the children and families you work with?

REFLECTIVE TASK

Use Table 5.2 to identify key aspects in the case study of creativity being used as a therapeutic tool.

Table 5.2 Evidence of aspects of creativity found in the case study and the benefits of them

Aspects of creative approaches	Evidence for this in the case study	How this was beneficial
The therapist making a safe space Identifying emotions as a way to begin processing the trauma and build resilience A Common Third activity The three Ps Any other creative activities		

Conclusion

In this chapter we have explored how various aspects of creativity can be utilised to help others process and heal from mind trauma, anger, grief and adversity. We considered how to foster appropriate relationships and activities, what action might be taken if things go wrong and the importance of allowing children and families to process trauma and its accompanying emotions at their own pace and in an informed, intentional way. Thus, creativity is more than high arts and entertainment, but when used as a therapeutic tool can bring healing and hope to many.

Creativity: key points

- For something to be considered creative it should be imaginative, purposeful, original and valuable (NAACEE, 1999)
- There are many developmental, social and health benefits to engaging in creative activities (Cultural Learning Alliance, 2017)
- Creative activities can aid in processing trauma (Parker, 2020)
- Attachments between parents and children can be fostered through creative activities such as art and music
- Engaging with music can release the mood enhancing chemical dopamine (Zaatar et al., 2023). Group musical activities can support a sense of belonging, increased confidence and self-esteem (Wood et al., 2013).
- Being creative can induce a state of flow (Karkou et al., 2023), which improves mood, increases confidence and overall life satisfaction (Parsons et al., 2023).
- Engaging in role play and drama can facilitate resilience by temporarily imposing an internal locus of control, releasing the child from emotional baggage and exploring unprocessed issues in a detached way.
- Art activities are useful for children with mild trauma, providing a safe space to express difficult emotions (Gordon, 2007).
- Appleton's (2001) Avenues of Hope maintained that trauma-experienced children transition through four stages: impact, retreat, acknowledgement and reconstruction as part of their journey to resolution.

- Creating a safe and nurturing space is a key aspect of healing from trauma (Mutch & Latai, 2019) and needs careful consideration.
- The social pedagogy concept of the three Ps (professional, personal and private) is a useful framework for establishing warm relationships.
- Common Third activities, where the focus is on a joint activity, can enable trusting relationships to naturally develop.
- Teamwork and reflective practice are important for working effectively with children (Parker, 2020).
- Trauma-experienced children must be allowed to go through the pain of an unmet stage of development to enable growth (Robbins, 2001, cited in Parker, 2020).
- The child needs to know that you can bear their pain and will not shrink away (Parker, 2020).

ADDITIONAL RESOURCES

- Curtis, E. (2022) *Art therapy activities for kids: 75 evidence-based art projects to improve behavior, build social skills, and boost emotional resilience.* Oakland, CA: Callisto Kids.

This is a very accessible book with easy, creative activities to help children identify and express emotions.

- Treisman, K. (2017) *A therapeutic treasure box for working with children and adolescents with developmental trauma: creative techniques and activities.* London: Jessica Kingsley Publishers

This jam-packed book has lots of creative, evidence-based ideas for working with trauma-experienced children and young people.

References

Appleton, V. (2001) Avenues of Hope: art therapy and the resolution of trauma. *Journal of the American Art Therapy Association*, 18(1): 6-13. doi: 10.1080/07421656.2001.10129454.

Armstrong, V.G. and Ross, J. (2022) The experiences of parents and infants using home-based art intervention aimed at improving wellbeing and connectedness in their relationships, *Frontiers in Psychology*, 13(732562), pp.1-14.

Bang, A.H. (2016) The restorative and transformative power of the arts in conflict resolution. *Journal of Transformative Education*, 14(4), pp. 355-376. doi:10.1177/1541344616655886

Belsky, J. and Fearon, R.M. (2002) Early attachment security, subsequent maternal sensitivity, and later child development: does continuity in development depend upon continuity of caregiving? *Attachment and Human Development*, 4(3), pp. 361-387. doi:10.1080/14616730210167267.

Bigelow, A.E., MacLean, K., Proctor, J., Myatt, T., Gillis, R. and Power, M. (2010) Maternal sensitivity throughout infancy: continuity and relation to attachment security. *Infant Behavior and Development*, 33(6), pp. 50-60. doi: 10.1016/j.infbeh.2009. 10.009

Bruce, D. and Hackett, S. (2021) Developing art therapy practice within perinatal parent-infant mental health. *International Journal of Art Therapy*, 26(3), pp. 111-122. doi: https://doi.org/10.1080/17454832.2020.1801784.

Camic, P.M. (2008) Playing in the mud: health psychology, the arts and creative approaches to health care. *Journal of Health Psychology*, 13(2), pp. 287-298. doi: 10.1177/1359105307086698.

Casement, P.J. (1985) *Learning from the patient*. London: The Guilford Press.

Chambers, H. and Petrie, P. (2009). *A learning framework for artist pedagogues*. London: Creativity, Culture and Education and National Children's Bureau. Available at: https://www.a-n.co.uk/research/a-learning-framework-for-artist-pedagogues (Accessed 1 September 2024).

Christiansen, J., Qualter, P., Friis K. Pedersen, S.S., Lund, R., Andersen, C.M., Bekker-Jeppesen, M. and Lasgaard, M. (2021) Associations of loneliness and social isolation with physical and mental health among adolescents and young adults, *Perspectives in Public Health*, 141(4), pp. 226-236. doi: 10.1177/17579139211016077.

Craft, A., Jeffrey, B. and Leibling, M. (eds.) (2001) *Creativity in education*. London: Continuum Publishing.

Csikszentmihalyi, M. (1990) *Flow: the psychology of optimal experience*. New York: Harper & Row.

Cultural Learning Alliance (2017) *Key research findings; the case for cultural learning*. Available at: https://www.culturallearningalliance.org.uk/wp-content/uploads/2024/01/CLA-key-findings-2017.pdf (Accessed 29 August 2024).

Davies, S.M., Silverio, S.A., Christiansen, P. and Fallon, V. (2021) Maternal infant bonding and perceptions of infant temperament: the mediating role of maternal mental health, *Journal of Affective Disorders*, 282(March), pp. 1323-1329. doi:10.1016/j. jad.2021.01.023.

Deci, E.L., and Ryan, R.M. (2000) The 'What' and 'Why' of goal pursuits: human needs and the self determination of behavior. *Psychological Inquiry*, 11(4), pp. 227-268. doi: 10.1207/S15327965PLI1104_01.

Folostinaa, R., Tudorachea, L., Michela, T., Erzsebeta, B., Agheanaa, V. and Hocaoglua, H. (2015) Using play and drama in developing resilience in children at risk. *Procedia – Social and Behavioral Sciences*, 197, pp. 2362-2368. doi: 10.1016/j.sbspro.2015.07.283.

Gibbs, L., Mutch, C., MacDougall, C. and O'Connor, P. (2013) Research with, by, for, and about children: lessons from disaster contexts, *Global Studies of Childhood*, 5(3), pp. 129-141.

Gillies, D., Taylor, F., Gray C, O'Brien, L., and D'Abrew, N. (2013) Psychological therapies for the treatment of post-traumatic stress disorder in children and adolescents (Review), *Evidence-Based Child Health*, 8(3), pp. 1004-1116. doi:10.1002/ebch.1916. PMID: 23877914.

Gordon, R. (2007) Thirty years of trauma work: clarifying and broadening the consequences of trauma. *Psychotherapy in Australia*, 13(3), pp. 12-19.

Hasley, K., Jones, M. and Lord, P. (2006) *What works in stimulating creativity in socially excluded young people*. Slough: National Foundation for Educational Research. Available at: https://www.nfer.ac.uk/media/ln3ee44k/nes01.pdf (Accessed 29 August 2024).

Humphrey, R. (2020). Social pedagogy, music making and adopted children. *International Journal of Social Pedagogy*, 9(1), pp. 1-8. doi:https://doi.org/10.14324/111.444.ijsp.2020.v9.x.007.

Karkou, V., Omylinska-Thurston, J., Parsons, A., Nair, K., Starkey, J., Haslam, S.,Thurston, S. and Marshall, L. D. (2022) Bringing creative psychotherapies to primary NHS mental health services in the UK: a feasibility study on patient and staff experiences of Arts for the Blues workshops delivered at improving access to psychological therapies (IAPT) services. *Counselling and Psychotherapy Research*, 22(3), pp. 616-628. doi: https://doi.org/10.1002/capr.12544

Kasca, M. (2015) *Social pedagogy, an invitation*. London: Jacaranda Development.

Macdonald, D., Han, J., Elder, E. and Boydell, K.M. (2023) Parents' perspectives of an arts engagement program supporting children with anxiety, *International Journal of Environmental Research and Public Health*, 20(18), p. 6771. doi:10.3390/ijerph20186771.

Meins, E., Fernyhough, C., Fradley, E. and Tuckey, M. (2001). Rethinking maternal sensitivity: mothers' comments on infants' mental processes predict security of attachment at 12 months, *Journal of. Child Psychology and Psychiatry and Allied Disciplines*, 42(5), pp. 637-648. doi:10.1111/1469-7610. 00759.

Mutch, C. and Latai, L. (2019) Creativity beyond the formal curriculum: arts-based interventions in post-disaster trauma settings, *Pastoral Care in Education*, 37(3), pp. 230-256. doi: 10.1080/02643944.2019.1642948

National Advisory Committee on Creative and Cultural Education (NACCCE) (1999) *All our futures: creativity, culture and education*. London: DFEE. Available at: https://sirkenrobinson.com/pdf/allourfutures.pdf (Accessed 29.8.2024).

Ogińska-Bulik, N. and Kobylarczyk, M. (2015) Resiliency and social support as factors promoting the process of resilience in adolescents—wards of children's homes. *Health Psychology Report*, 3(3), pp. 210- 219. doi: https://doi.org/10.5114/hpr.2015.49045.

Orr, P. (2007) Art therapy with children after a disaster: a content analysis. *The Arts in Psychotherapy*, 34(4), pp. 350-361.

Parker, C. (2020) Creative mentoring: a creative response to promote learning and wellbeing with children in care. A service developed by Derbyshire County Council's virtual school. *International Journal of Social Pedagogy*, 9(1), pp. 9-18.

Parsons, A., Dubrow-Marshall, L., Turner R., Thurston, S., Starkey, J., Omylinska-Thurston, J. and Karkou, V. (2023) The importance of psychological flow in a creative, embodied and enactive psychological therapy approach (Arts for the Blues), *Body, Movement and Dance in Psychotherapy*, 18(2), pp. 137-154. doi:10.1080/17432979.2022.2130431

Pawlicka, P. and Kaźmierczak, M. (2018) Between emotions and cognition: exploring the concept of resilience, in Russell, W. and Schuur, K. (eds.) *The strength of European diversity for building children's resilience through play and drama: a collection of articles from the EU Erasmus Plus ARTPAD project 2015-2018*. Gloucester: University of Gloucestershire, pp. 17-20.

Pietromonaco, P.R. and Powers, S.I. (2015) Attachment and health-related physiological stress processes, *Current Opinion in Psychology*, 1(1), pp. 34-39. doi:10.1016/j.copsyc.2014.12.001.

Rotter, J.B. (1966) Generalized expectancies for internal versus external control of reinforcement, *Psychological Monographs*, 80 (Whole No. 609). Available at: https://www.neshaminy.org/site/handlers/filedownload.ashx?moduleinstanceid=34376&dataid=51132&FileName=Article%207-Are%20You%20the%20Master%20of%20Your%20Fate.pdf (Accessed 4 September 2024).

Russell, W. (2018) 'Thinking a little differently about resilience and play', in W. Russell and K. Schuur (eds). *The strength of European diversity for building children's resilience through play and drama: a collection of articles from the EU Erasmus Plus ARTPAD project 2015-2018*, Gloucester: University of Gloucestershire, pp. 92-98.

Ryan, R.M. and Deci, E.L. (2000) Self-determination theory and the facilitation of intrinsic motivation, social development and wellbeing, *American Psychologist*, 55(4, pp. 68-78.

Sawyer, R.K. (2015) Drama, theatre and performance creativity, in Davis, S., Ferholt, B., Grainger Clemson, H., Jansson, S.-M. and Marjanovic-Shane, A. (eds.) *Dramatic interactions in education: Vygotskian and sociocultural approaches to drama, education and research*. London: Bloomsbury, pp. 245-260.

Sellers, R. (2020) *Redefining trauma*. Available at: https://www.rachelesellers.com/blog/redefining-trauma (Accessed 8 September 2024).

Stern, D.N. (1985) *The interpersonal world of the infant: a view from psychoanalysis and developmental psychology*. New York: Basic Books.

Tait, N. and Reilly, M. (2021) *CORC report: drawing and talking*. Child Outcomes Research Consortium. Available at: https://25717290.fs1.hubspotusercontent-eu1.net/hubfs/25717290/DT%20Blog/pdf-files/CORC-Report-Drawing-and-Talking_.pdf (Accessed 16 December 2025).

Tugade, M.M. and Fredrickson, B.L. (2004) Resilient individuals use positive emotions to bounce back from negative emotional experiences. *Journal of Personality and Social Psychology*, 86(2), pp. 320-333. doi: 10.1037/0022-3514.86.2.320.

Vansteenkiste, M., Ryan, R.M. and Soenens, B. (2020) Basic psychological need theory: advancements, critical themes, and future directions. *Motivation and Emotion*, 44(1), pp. 1-31. doi: https://doi.org/10.1007/s11031-019-09818-1.

Wood, L., Ivery, P., Donovan, R. and Lambin, E. (2013) "To the beat of a different drum": improving the social and mental wellbeing of at-risk young people through drumming. *Journal of Public Mental Health*, 12(2), pp. 70-79. doi: 10.1108/JPMH-09-2012-0002. Available at: https://www.researchgate.net/publication/253650817_To_the_beat_of_a_different_drum_Improving_the_social_and_mental_wellbeing_of_at-risk_young_people_through_drumming (Accessed 16 January 2025).

Wu, Y., Zhang, C., Liu, H., Duan, C., Li, C., Fan, J., Li, H., Chen, L., Xu, H., Li, X., Guo, Y., Wang, Y., Li, X., Li, J., Zhang, T., You, Y., Li, H., Yang, S., Tao, X., Xu, Y., Lao, H., Wen, M., Zhou, Y., Wang, J., Chen, Y., Meng, D., Zhai, J., Ye, Y., Zhong, Q., Yang, X., Zhang, D., Zhang, J., Wu, X., Chen, W., Dennis, C.L. and Huang, H.F. (2020) Perinatal depressive and anxiety symptoms of pregnant women during the coronavirus disease 2019 outbreak in China. *American Journal of Obstetrics and Gynecology*, 223(240), pp. e1-9. doi: 10.1016/j.ajog.2020.05.009.

Zaatar, M.T., Alhakim, K., Enayeh, M. and Tamer, R. (2023) The transformative power of music: insights into neuroplasticity, health, and disease. *Brain, Behavior, & Immunity - Health*, 12(35), pp. 1-11. doi: 10.1016/j.bbih.2023.100716.

6
The great outdoors

Introduction

When eating at a café on a warm, sunny day and given the option of sitting indoors or outdoors, people tend to choose outdoors. It is both relaxing and invigorating to breathe in fresh air, do a spot of people watching and take in the view. In this chapter we explore the many benefits of the great outdoors including why using it can be a powerful tool for those affected by trauma and adversity. We also consider inequalities in access to the outdoors and the danger of looking at children's experiences of it through rose-tinted spectacles.

The physical health benefits

Have you ever climbed to the top of a hill and been rewarded by the view of a stunning landscape for miles around? Unbeknown to you your eye muscles were getting a workout, being flexed in an increasingly rare way as we spend much of our time in closed-in spaces. People who spend more time in activities outdoors, however, have fewer incidents of myopia (a condition that makes distant objects appear blurry) (Rose et al., 2008). Evidence also suggests that outdoor activity increases vitamin D absorption, essential for bone, teeth and muscle health, (McCurdy et al., 2010), and the development of the vestibular and proprioceptive systems (Hanscom, 2016), i.e., a sense of balance and knowing where your body is in space – key to all other senses. When children hurtle down a hill, for example, their heads are moving in a different way than when upright, and the moving fluid in the head stimulates hair growth (Hanscom, 2016).

The past 20 years has seen a worrying increase in the number of children having sleeping difficulties, experiencing gastric anxiety and poor wellbeing (Liu et al., 2022), yet a 2006 study found that spending time in natural environments helped counteract these symptoms (Frost, 2006).

The benefits of risky play in the outdoor environment

Risky play is defined by Sandseter as "thrilling and exciting forms of physical play that involve uncertainty and a risk of physical injury" (Sandseter, 2010, p.67), and despite adult endeavours to limit children's risky play, the drive to engage in it when given a free choice persists

(Sandseter & Kennair, 2011; Sandseter et al., 2021). Risky play was also discussed in Chapter 4 but, to summarise, evidence suggests that risky play, particularly in the outdoors, enables children to push boundaries and test their limits, and is exciting and stimulating (Sandseter, 2010). Examples include exploring the four natural elements (fire, wind, water and earth), rough and tumble play, play with tools and opportunities to "disappear" (Andrews, 2012, p.14).

The outdoor environment is particularly suitable for risky play because of the prevalence of "loose parts" (Nicholson, 1971) that provide opportunities for discovery, creativity and combinatorial flexibility (Hughes, 2001, p.38), the bringing together of past experiences, knowledge and available resources to solve a problem in a new way. This implies a particular type of outdoor environment, one with "multiple affordances" (Gibson, 1996, p.133) that invite a variety of uses for an object, for example, a long stick can form part of a shelter, be a divider of territory or become a magic wand. An expanse of grass with no variation in height, nowhere to dig, swing, balance or hide, no sand, water, rocks or branches will offer little challenge or risk. When natural spaces are dynamic and diverse however, there are opportunities for children to experience a profound sense of wellbeing and flow, where concentration and engagement are at their peak (Csikszentmihalyi, 2013) (see Chapter 5 for more on flow).

The holistic benefits

We often imagine that when children are outdoors, they are energetic, even dizzy, however, they also need downtime to recuperate and prevent over-stimulation. This can be problematic if children's outdoor play is framed as part of an obesity reduction, agenda, and the more sedate interactions with nature disregarded (Alexander et al., 2014). The restorative benefits of engaging with the outdoors was confirmed when I (Nicola) undertook primary research to determine how and where children enjoyed playing. One child responded, "I like to be left alone with my thoughts and just wander around" (Stobbs, 2024). This implies that Csikszentmihalyi's concept of flow is found in many forms when children engage with the outdoor environment, for example, observable outer behaviour and the inner peaceful feelings. Alexander et al.'s (2014) interview with a child about their favourite activity similarly revealed that children's physical actions do not always equate with their inner thoughts,

> Not sure I mentioned this, but it's the swings . . . they allow me to let my thoughts take off and run free and allow me to empty my mind and to relax. I really like that. Often, I go to the park next to the school, and I always take the same swing, facing a big tree, lots of sky…. I really do like swinging. One time I went to the park, and I stayed for an hour, swinging the whole time…. I can think of things. Sometimes what I think about is actually drawing.
>
> (p.1336)

The authors note that the child speaks differently about their time on the swings and the time spent at sports practice; the first is intrinsic and relaxing, the second is motivated by extrinsic obligations (Nielsen & Hansen, 2007). While we can observe and measure physical development when children are active, we should be aware that there is likely to be an inner dialogue that accompanies it as children learn about themselves: "Am I brave enough to walk across the log over the river?" "How high can I climb?" "Why does my heart pound when I run?" (Hewes, 2006, p.4).

Critical questions

1. Have you ever felt the better after spending time outdoors? If so, how could you explain this effect?
2. What are the advantages and disadvantages of attempting to measure the benefits of being outdoors?
3. What does a focus on instrumental aspects of engaging with the outdoors indicate about adults' expressions of value?

Forest School

One approach combining measurable learning and the holistic benefits of being outdoors is Forest School. This initiative originated in Nordic countries and has grown in popularity in the United Kingdom since the end of the twentieth century. The key principles of Forest School are:

- Forest School is a long-term process of frequent and regular sessions in a woodland or natural environment, rather than a one-off visit. Planning, adaptation, observations and reviewing are integral elements of Forest School
- Forest School takes place in a woodland or natural wooded environment to support the development of a relationship between the learner and the natural world
- Forest School aims to promote the holistic development of all those involved, fostering resilient, confident, independent and creative learners
- Forest School offers learners the opportunity to take supported risks appropriate to the environment and themselves
- Forest School is run by qualified Forest School practitioners who continuously maintain and develop their professional practice
- Forest School uses a range of learner-centred processes to create a community for development and learning

(Forest School Association, 2018)

Although there are still timetabled lessons with measurable curriculum outcomes as there would be inside the classroom, Forest School takes a different approach, for example, when children build shelters, they use creativity and imagination, mathematical and problem-solving skills, they listen and give instructions to others, articulate their thoughts, and build resilience and perseverance.

Forest School is flexible and responsive to group needs, for example, an Australian school replaced the term Forest School with Bush School, reflecting a more authentic application to their context (Cumming & Nash, 2015). Researchers have suggested that one of its strengths is its openness to social construction in this way (Leather, 2018) because expectations of how to engage with spaces are often culturally dependent. Unusual spaces, particularly wild spaces, may disrupt these cultural norms because each child or adult experiences or interprets them in their own way. Waite and Pratt (2009) propose that the outdoors can enable transformative learning that transcends culture, for example, not waiting to be told what to do by a teacher.

 Case study – Forest School leader

Sarah Watkins is an author, presenter, Forest School leader and university lecturer. Here Sarah writes about an experience she had as a Forest School leader.

> I had the privilege of running a long-term project which immersed trauma- experienced children in the outdoors. One child, Kay, was a five-year-old Sudanese refugee. She and her family were forcibly displaced from their home and travelled to England via Greece.
>
> Kay was softly spoken and shy. She seemed withdrawn in our first session and was initially reluctant to join in toasting s'mores over the campfire. She watched the others carefully. One of the key things for us was to show the children that this is a safe space where they can take risks, physically and emotionally, with our support.
>
> Kay enjoyed touching pieces of fabric, especially gold, glittery material. She would drape it over her knees, sitting in the shade of a tree, smiling.
>
> As the sessions progressed, Kay started to speak. At the end of one session, she hugged me and whispered, "Thank you!"
>
> As she gained confidence, Kay began to try activities such as bug hunting and swinging in the hammock. We never pressurised her but let her explore at her own pace.
>
> During one session, Kay said quietly, "I love Dandy Lions!" In another, she said, "Marshmallows please!" Requesting something was a big step for Kay.
>
> As the weeks went by, Kay was visibly more excited to walk over to the outdoor area, a quiet, smiling child in a group of exuberant children. We began to hear her laugh and become absorbed in activities like drilling wood, hammering and fire lighting.
>
> At the end of the project, we asked the children to reflect on their time with us. Kay told us her favourite part was "being in the group". This made me look again at Kay's participation outdoors. For Kay, being able to be with the group in her own way, doing things at her own pace and choosing when to contribute was the best thing about coming to our wild outdoor space. This project was funded by a family who have faced tragedy by committing to help others. Laura Price set up George's Fund to remember her five-year- old son George who died of a brain tumour in 2020. Laura explains, "As a mum, your jobs is to tell your children that 'everything will be ok'. I couldn't do that for George, so if we can make a small difference to another child's life then it will give us huge comfort."

Critical questions

1. Can you identify the key principles of Forest School in this case study?
2. How did Kay progress as part of this experience?
3. Why would it be difficult to track this on a traditional developmental/achievement chart?
4. In your opinion, what was key to Kay's progress?

The practice vignette below explores the power of outdoor learning for children in inner-city environments.

Practice vignette

Abish is a teacher working in an inner-city school. She takes the children in her class to a local environmental centre with a small wood. The children are given free time to explore, and Abish enjoys hearing their delight as they gather sticks and conkers, climb over tree stumps and build dens.

One child, Izzy, excitedly exclaims, "I've just seen a tree with apples growing on it!" Puzzled at why this is so exciting, Abish responds, "That's nice, but you knew that apples grow on trees, didn't you?" to which Izzy replied, "Yes, but I've never seen them in real life!"

The experience changed Izzy in a small way, her previous knowledge of apples had come from the theoretical study of apples, but her thrill at happening upon actual growing apples suggests that some learning is quantifiably different. It is experienced emotionally in a way that enhances intellectual knowledge (Waite & Pratt, 2009). This does not diminish cognitive learning but underlines the complexity of learning and invites us to consider *where* children learn as well as *what* they learn (Waite & Pratt, 2009). No matter how well written a textbook or how articulate a teacher, some knowledge can only be acquired through real-life experiences.

Critical question

Do you agree that the outdoors offers opportunities for 'transformative learning'? Why?

Nature as a retreat

As has been outlined, children derive many benefits from playing outdoors (O'Brien & Murray, 2007). If we look beyond the instrumental factors, however, there may be a more primitive, (i.e., not conscious) reason why playing outdoors is such a draw for children.

I remember as a child being released from the classroom for 'playtime', running with my friends to the small woodland at the bottom of the school playing field. Accessing it through a broken wall only made it more exciting, out of reach of teachers and far away from tedious schoolwork. In her book, *Secret Spaces of Childhood* (2010) Elizabeth Goodenough depicts how children have always played outdoors in this way, building dens, climbing trees, digging holes and tunnels, finding secret places for play, which are often used as a retreat from worries and difficult memories. The desire to be away from adults in hidden environments with friends fulfils a longing for ownership, freedom and control over a life that is generally directed by adults (Lester & Maudsley, 2006). The seclusion of the space is an important part of its appeal; being on the perimeter of boundaries offers peace and quiet, leading Dyment *et al.* (2009) to suggest that this enables children to feel empowered, acting as social agents over their environment rather than succumbing to feelings of helplessness. For me, the joy of escaping to the woods in school playtime offered mental respite from concentrating on grammatical rules and mathematical equations. For children with more serious issues, such as stressful home lives or relationships, deliberately choosing to be outside and away from humans can provide welcome relief (Bingley & Milligan, 2004). Allowing children to spend time in the outdoors is essential for tension release, whether from everyday cares or more serious abuse and neglect (Korpela *et al.*, 2001).

Children's instinct to build dens and shelters has led to a suggestion that this is a rehearsal for leaving home, creating a separate, new home from materials found in the natural world, based on the experience of their current home (Sobel, 1993). Children's need to create a refuge may be an evolutionary characteristic found in all humans, where they can watch without being seen, particularly where there is a potential threat or danger (Orians & Heerwagen, 1992). The evident enjoyment children experience when engaging in outdoor survival games such as shelter making, capture the flag and hide and seek suggests that they find innate satisfaction from these activities (Pyle, 2002).

Attachment to place

The long-lasting benefits of a secure attachment to family and friends are well documented (Bowlby, 1969, 1973; Ainsworth & Bell, 1970) and discussed in Chapter 3, but the benefits of an emotional attachment to a place should not be overlooked (Bird, 2007). Attachment to a place comes when people feel strengthened and renewed from being in that place, contributing to a strong personal identity in relation to a physical environment (Bird, 2007). Given that the natural, outdoor environment is consistently reported to be a preferred place for positive mental health (Stewart & Eccleston, 2020) its therapeutic potential should not be missed.

The outdoor environment is unique because it is experienced as both a public and a private space. I know, for example, that a favourite tree on the walk to school is not mine alone, yet I have watched it change through the seasons, stopped to rest and recuperate under it, perhaps even climbed it, I feel a personal, emotional connection each time I pass by, recalling its significance in my life, content that it is available when I need it. In that sense, it is mine. If I see others sitting under 'my' tree, I experience a shared identification with my neighbours and the local environment, the tree is now 'ours', which contributes to group identity and encourages us to care for our community (Bow & Buys, 2003). The tree takes on "symbolic importance ... as a repository of emotions and relationships that give meaning and purpose to life" (Williams & Vaske, 2002 p.831). This is particularly the case when special places in the outdoors are enjoyed throughout generations. Connections are formed through shared experiences in the natural environment and can transcend time (Factor, 2004). I have fond memories as a little girl of running down sand dunes to splash in the sea during a day out with my granny, knowing that she enjoyed the same beach as a child. Even though my granny has now died I feel close to her when I visit the beach that we shared; being there softens my grief and reminds me that I am worthy of love.

In addition, when we have sorrow in our lives, visiting a natural environment that is meaningful to us can give a sense of constancy and steadiness that enables us to put troubles into perspective (Factor, 2004).

The outdoors and attention restoration

> [T]he enjoyment of scenery employs the mind without fatigue and yet exercises it, tranquilizes it and yet enlivens it; and thus, through the influence of the mind over the body, gives the effect of refreshing rest and reinvigoration to the whole system.
>
> (Olmstead, 1865)

As can be seen from this delightful quote from 1865, people have been instinctively drawn to nature for centuries. Rapid technological advancements in the 1980s resulted in a change in play patterns whereby children spent more time indoors and researchers started to wonder if this was harmful. Stephen and Rachel Kaplan were key researchers in this field and developed Attention Restoration Theory (ART) (Kaplan & Kaplan, 1989). ART proposes that in addition to bringing us pleasure, being outside in nature is restorative to our wellbeing and improves concentration levels (Ohly et al., 2016).

The Kaplans theorised that a restorative environment consists of four criteria:

1. **Being away** from our daily routines and worries in a physically separate environment (this might be a place within a place, for example, at home in a garden but away from energy draining tasks).
2. **Extent:** the environment should consist of familiar features that are interesting and stimulating.
3. **Fascination:** our attention is held without effort on our part, we no longer need to expend energy blocking out distractions. 'Fascination' is divided into two sections, hard and soft. Hard fascinations absorb us by taking all our attention, such as playing a racing game on a console. Soft fascinations are less stimulating, gardening, perhaps. Both have their place; hard fascinations reduce boredom; soft fascinations offer time for reflection.
4. **Compatibility:** we should feel at ease, engaging with activities because we are intrinsically motivated to do so.

Applying these criteria helps us determine whether an environment has the potential to be restorative. When we spend too long on important but uninteresting activities requiring our full attention, maybe, following multi-step instructions for the construction of flat-pack furniture, we must block out interesting, but less important activities to avoid making errors. Continually resisting this pull of distraction can be exhausting but being in environments that naturally hold our attention can offset this. These are known as restorative environments because they reduce tension and restore calm to our brains, enabling us to return renewed to our original task.

Being in the natural world meets all these criteria to a certain degree: we leave our daily routines (being away), when walking in the outdoors we can follow pathways that have both familiar elements (for example, trees and grass) and lead to different routes and destinations (extent), providing a variety of natural features such as plants and wildlife to see on the way (fascination). Additionally, spending time in nature allows opportunities to reflect on unresolved issues and life goals (Kaplan & Berman, 2010).

Some of the most significant findings of ART for those working with children and families in a therapeutic way relate to Attention Deficit Hyperactivity Disorder (ADHD), mental fatigue and stress recovery.

ADHD

Recognisable symptoms of ADHD are demonstrated by two behaviour types: (1) difficulty concentrating, short attention spans, losing things and making frequent mistakes, and (2) hyperactivity and impulsiveness, for example, constant fidgeting, being unable to keep quiet and little sense of danger (NHS, n.d.).

Research in 2011 to determine whether there were any links between children's declining time spent in nature and the increasing prevalence of ADHD diagnosis (van den Berg & van den Berg, 2011) found that children attending a school for children with ADHD performed better on a task requiring sustained concentration after a trip to the woods compared to a trip to a town where they completed a similar task. The children's behaviour was also more sociable and less aggressive in the woods than in the town.

A further study undertaken in 2014 found that students diagnosed with ADHD who took 20-minute walks in either urban or natural environments found the natural environments were significantly more restorative than the urban environment (Thal, 2014).

Mental fatigue

A study by Hartig *et al.*, (1991) compared two groups sent on a backpacking holiday, one in the wilderness and one in a more urban environment. Emotional regulation, cognitive performance and physiological measures, for example, heart rate and muscle tension, were restored after spending time in nature, but the performance of the group holidaying in the urban environment was worse than it had been before the holiday.

Another study found that you do not even need to be in natural environments to enjoy the restorative benefits. Berto (2005) gave three sets of participants a direct attention, mentally fatiguing task. She then showed each group different photographs, one of geometric shapes, another of restorative environments and the final group of non-restorative environments. The groups then completed another direct attention task and those who had looked at the restorative photographs performed better. The effects were replicated using video images of natural environments (Wang *et al.*, 2016).

Stress recovery

Everyone has daily stress, an unexpected delay to a meeting, or too many demands in the time available. Prolonged stress, however, can cause debilitating symptoms such as jumping to conclusions, tunnel vision, catastrophising, casting blame (either internally or externally), overgeneralising and unhelpful emotional reasoning (e.g., overreacting) (Boniwell & Tunairiu, 2019). One of the most stressful situations is being treated for cancer and a study by Cimprich (1993) found that breast cancer patients who spent time in natural environments were less stressed, more likely to return to work and had a higher quality of life than those who had not. A later study had similar results, and the authors proposed that virtual reality headsets could enable bedbound patients to benefit from an immersive experience in the natural world (Song *et al.*, 2022).

Although some areas of ART are subject to criticism, for example, there are no studies measuring the long-term effects of ART, it is nevertheless a theory worth considering when working therapeutically with children and families. Problems such as crime, violence and the anxiety associated with poverty and financial worries are often predominant in poorer neighbourhoods. Exposing those living in these areas to more natural environments could help mitigate some of these anxieties by providing restoration and recovery from the mental fatigue of constantly thinking about difficult situations. As well as tackling these issues from a social angle, taking an environmental perspective may also prove effective.

REFLECTIVE TASK

Reflect on the questions posed and complete Table 6.1 relating to the many benefits of being in the outdoors.

Table 6.1 Reflection on the benefits of the outdoors

What games and activities did you play outdoors as a child?
How has this affected your attitude to being outdoors?
Have you ever experienced comfort and stress relief from being outdoors?
Have you felt an attachment to a certain place outdoors?
How might playing and learning outdoors enable children to feel capable in a way that they may not feel in the classroom?
Is children's access to the outdoors restricted? Explain your answer.
Should parents dictate whether their child should spend time in the outdoors or not? Why?

Challenging the romanticised view of an outdoor childhood

While spending time in nature has therapeutic benefits, we should refrain from indulging in an overly romanticised view of childhood and nature, oversimplifying the complexity of children's lives and the uniqueness of every family context. Lester and Maudsley (2006) explain that a discourse of the 'natural child', imagined as carefree and healthy, with freedom to enjoy the natural world, risks 'othering' children in ways that that do not match with their lived reality (Atken, 2001). Children in rural locations are rarely allowed to roam freely over farmers' fields and can live far away from friends (Lester & Maudsley, 2006). Those from ethnic minority backgrounds also have complex relationships with natural environments (Morris, 2003), as do children with disabilities (Horton, 2017).

Children will, however, make the best of things even in less than idyllic settings. In urban areas they find 'in-between spaces' to play (Aminpour *et al.*, 2020) such as under stairs, walkways and small, contained enclosures. They do not need to be in nature to be fun. As children spend less time in nature, however, there is a risk of disengagement. Researchers from the University of Cambridge found that eight-year-olds were able to identify more Pokémon characters than wildlife (Balmford *et al.*, 2002) suggesting that children do not lack learning capacity, but fantasy worlds are becoming more engaging than the natural world. It falls to practitioners to appreciate the therapeutic benefits of the outdoor environment and share this with children and families.

Conclusion

In this chapter we began by considered the more measurable benefits of the outdoor environment on health, wellbeing and development. We reflected on the advantages of risk in play and how Forest School offers children unique opportunities for self-discovery and healing as well as curriculum learning. We took this further and considered other therapeutic benefits, such as the use of outdoors as a retreat, and how a sense of place can offer a secure attachment similar to the caregiver bond. We discussed Attention Restoration Theory and outlined the four criteria that make an environment restorative, concluding that the natural world has the potential to meet all these measures. We explained how this is of particular interest to those working in the fields of ADHD, mental fatigue and stress recovery. It also invited us, however, to trouble an over-simplified discourse of childhood and the accessibility of the outdoors for all. Finally, it called on practitioners to promote the special benefits of the great outdoors before these are lost.

The great outdoors: key points

- Physical health benefits from spending time outdoors include fewer incidents of myopia, increased vitamin D absorption and the development of the vestibular and proprioceptive systems.
- Risky play is particularly suited to the outdoor environment due to the prevalence of loose parts (Nicholson, 1971) and opportunities for combinatorial flexibility (Hughes, 2001). The dynamic yet tranquil characteristics of outdoor settings are conducive to the experience of flow (Csikszentmihalyi, 2013).
- When children engage with the outdoor environment there are holistic benefits that may not be discernible from their outward behaviour.
- Forest School utilises outdoor resources for curriculum objectives potentially leading to new understanding and transformative learning.
- Children use nature as a retreat from difficult situations and to assert control, for example, to practise leaving home and responding to danger or threat (Orians & Heerwagen, 1992).
- Having an attachment to an outdoor environment contributes to a personal and group identity (Bow & Buys, 2003) that enhances life (Williams & Vaske, 2002 p.831), particularly when it is shared by different generations (Factor, 2004).
- Attention Restoration Theory (Kaplan & Kaplan, 1989) proposes that being in natural environments improves mental health and concentration (Ohly *et al.*, 2016).
- A restorative environment consists of four components: being away, extent, fascination and compatibility. Being in the natural world has the potential to meet all these criteria.
- The findings are particularly significant in the areas of ADHD, mental fatigue and stress recovery.
- Not all children have equal access to the natural world.

ADDITIONAL RESOURCES

- Woodland Trust Outdoor Learning Pack

This pack has tips and ideas for practitioners wanting to take learning outside the classroom. Available at: https://www.woodlandtrust.org.uk/media/43645/outdoor-learning-resource-pack.pdf (Accessed 23 August 2024).

- Harper, H.J., Rose, K. and Degal, D. (2019) *Nature-based therapy: a practitioner's guide to working outside with children, youth and families*. Gabriola, BC: New Society Publications.

An accessible, research-informed framework for using therapeutic approaches outside.

References

Ainsworth, M.D. and Bell, S.M. (1970) Attachment, exploration, and separation: illustrated by the behavior of one-year-olds in a strange situation, *Child Development*, 41(1), pp. 49–67. doi: https://doi.org/10.2307/1127388.

Alexander, S.A., Frohlich, K.L. and Fusco, C. (2014) Problematizing "play-for-health" discourses through children's photo-elicited narratives, *Qualitative Health Research*, 24(10), pp. 1329–1341.

Aminpour, F., Bishop, K. and Corkery, L. (2020) The hidden value of in-between spaces for children's self-directed play within outdoor school environments, *Landscape and Urban Planning*, 194, pp. 1–16.

Andrews, M. (2012) *Exploring play for early childhood studies*. London: Sage.

Atken, S.C. (2001) *Geographies of young people*. London: Routledge.

Balmford, A., Clegg, L., Coulson, T. and Taylor, J. (2002). Why conservationists should heed Pokémon, *Science*, 295(5564), pp. 1–2. doi: 10.1126/science.295.5564.2367b.

Berto, R. (2005) Exposure to restorative environments helps restore attentional capacity, *Journal of Environmental Psychology*, 25(3), pp. 249–259.

Bird, W. (2007) Natural thinking: investigating the links between the natural environment, biodiversity and mental health. Sandy, Bedfordshire: RSPB. www.rspb.org.uk/health. Available at: https://www.centreforecotherapy.org.uk/wp-content/uploads/2021/07/Natural-Thinking-RSPB-report.pdf (Accessed 20 August 2024).

Boniwell, I. and Tunariu, A.D. (2019) *Positive psychology: theory, research and applications*. Maidenhead: McGraw-Hill Education.

Bow, V. and Buys, E. (2003) Sense of community and place attachment: the natural environment plays a vital role in developing a sense of community, in Buys, L., Lyddon, J. and Bradley, R. (eds.) *Social change in the 21st century: 2003 Conference Refereed Proceedings*. Brisbane: Centre for Social Change Research. School of Humanities and Human Services QUT, Australia, pp. 1–18. Available at: https://eprints.qut.edu.au/115/1/Bow%26Buys.pdf (Accessed 20 August 2024)

Bowlby, J. (1969) *Attachment and loss. Vol 1: Attachment*. New York: Basic Books.

Bowlby, J. (1973) *Attachment and loss. Vol. 2: Separation: anxiety and anger*. New York: Basic Books.

Cimprich, B. (1993) Development of an intervention to restore attention in cancer patients, *Cancer Nursing*, 16(2), pp. 83–92.

Csikszentmihalyi, M. (2013) *Flow: the psychology of optimal experience*. New York: Random House.

Cumming, F. and Nash, M. (2015) An Australian perspective of a Forest School: shaping a sense of place to support learning, *Journal of Adventure Education and Outdoor Learning*, 15(4), pp. 296–309.

Dyment, J.E., Bell, A.C. and Lucas, A.J. (2009) The relationship between school ground design and intensity of physical activity, *Children's Geographies*, 7(3), pp. 261–276. doi: https://doi.org/10.1080/14733280903024423.

Factor, J. (2004) Tree stumps, manhole covers and rubbish tins: the invisible play-lines of a primary school playground, *Childhood*, 11(2), pp. 142–154.

Forest School Association (2018) What is Forest School? Available at: https://www.forestschoolassociation.org/what-is-forest-school (Accessed 19 August 2024).

Frost, J. (2006) *The dissolution of children's outdoor play: causes and consequences, presented to The Value of Play: a forum on risk, recreation and children's health*, 31 May. Available at: /www.ipema.org/Documents/Common%20Good%20PDF.pdf.

Gibson, J.J. (1996) *The ecological approach to visual perception*. Mahwah, NJ: Lawrence Erlbaum.

Goodenough, E. (2010) *Secret spaces of childhood*. Ann Arbor: University of Michigan Press.

Hanscom, A.J. (2016) *Balanced and barefoot: how unrestricted outdoor play makes for strong, confident, and capable children*. Oakland, CA: Raincoast Books.

Hartig, T., Mang, M. and Evans, G. (1991) Restorative effects of natural environment experiences, *Environment and Behavior*, 23(1), pp. 3–26. doi: https://doi.org/10.1177/0013916591231001.

Hewes, J. (2006) *Let the children play: nature's answer to early learning*. Toronto: Early Childhood Learning Knowledge Centre. Available at: https://roam.macewan.ca:8443/server/api/core/bitstreams/9154ea7f-7a83-4908-8857-90e4f9c6c481/content (Accessed 23 August 2024).

Hughes, B. (2001) *Evolutionary playwork and reflective analytical practice*. London. Routledge.

Hughes, F.P. (2010) Children, *play and development*. 4th edn. London. Sage.

Horton, J. (2017) Disabilities, urban natures and children's outdoor play. *Social and Cultural Geography*, 18(8), pp. 1152–1174. doi: https://doi.org/10.1080/14649365.2016.1245772.

Kaplan, S. and Berman M.G. (2010) Directed attention as a common resource for executive functioning and self-regulation, *Perspectives on Psychological Science*, 5(1), pp. 43–57. doi: 10.1177/1745691609356784.

Kaplan, R. and Kaplan, S. (1989) The *experience of nature: a psychological perspective*. New York: Cambridge University Press.

Korpela, K.M., Hartig, T., Kaiser, F.G. and Fuhrer, U. (2001) Restorative experience and self-regulation in favorite places. *Environment and Behavior*, 33(4), 572–589. doi: https://doi-org.apollo.worc.ac.uk/10.1177/00139160121973133.

Leather, M. (2018) A critique of Forest School: something lost in translation, *Journal of Outdoor Education*, 21(1), pp. 5–18. London: Springer.

Lester, S. and Maudsley, M. (2006) *Play naturally, a review of children's natural play*. London: Children's Play Council. Available at: https://www.playday.org.uk/wp-content/uploads/2015/11/play_naturally_a_review_of_childrens_natural_play.pdf (Accessed 1 August 2024).

Liu, J., Ji, X., Pitt, S., Wang, G., Rovit, E., Lipman, T. and Jiang, F. (2024) Childhood sleep: physical, cognitive, and behavioral consequences and implications. *World Journal of Pediatrics*, 20(2), pp. 122–132. doi:10.1007/s12519-022-00647-w.

McCurdy, L.E., Winterbottom, K.E., Mehta, S.S. and Roberts, J.R. (2010) Using nature and outdoor activity to improve children's health, *Current Problems in Pediatric and Adolescent Health Care*, 40(5), pp. 102–117.

Milligan, C. and Bingley, A. (2004). *Climbing trees and building dens: mental health and wellbeing in young adults' long-term experience of childhood play experiences*. Institute for Health Research, University of Lancaster. Available at: https://www.research.lancs.ac.uk/portal/files/236475416/Climbing_trees_and_building_dens.pdf (Accessed 20 August 2024).

Morris, N. (2003) *Black and minority ethnic groups and public open spaces*. Edinburgh, OPENspace. Available at: https://www.openspace.eca.ed.ac.uk/wp-content/uploads/2015/10/Black-and-Minority-Ethnic-Groups-and-Public-Open-Space-literature-review.pdf (Accessed 23. August 2024).

NHS online (n.d.) Attention Deficit Hyperactivity Disorder (ADHD). Available at: https://www.nhs.uk/conditions/attention-deficit-hyperactivity-disorder-adhd/symptoms (Accessed 11 August 2024).

Nicholson, S. (1971) The Theory of Loose Parts – how not to cheat children, *Landscape Architecture Quarterly*, 62(1), pp. 30–34.

Nielsen, T. and Hansen, K.B. (2007) Do green areas affect health? Results from a Danish survey on the use of green areas and health indicators, *Health and Place*, 13(4), pp. 839–850.

O'Brien, L. and Murray, R., (2007) Forest School and its impacts on young children: case studies in Britain. *Urban Forestry and Urban Greening*, 6(4), pp. 249–265.

Ohly, H., White, M.P., Wheeler, B.W., Bethel, A., Ukoumunne, O.C., Nikolaou, V. and Garside, R. (2016) Attention Restoration Theory: a systematic review of the attention restoration potential of exposure to natural environments, *Journal of Toxicology and Environmental Health, Part B*, 19(7), pp. 305–343. doi: https://doi.org/10.1080/10937404.2016.1196155.

Olmstead, F.L. (1865) *Yosemite and the Mariposa Grove: a preliminary report, 1865*. Available at: www.yosemite.ca.us/library/olmsted/report.html (Accessed 21 August 2024).

Orians, G.H. and Heerwagen, J H. (1992) Evolved responses to landscapes, in Barkow, J. H. Cosmides, L. and Tooby, J. (eds.) *The adapted mind: evolutionary psychology and the generation of culture*. Oxford: Oxford University Press, pp. 555–579.

Pyle, R. (2002) Eden in a vacant lot: special places, species and kids in community of life, in Kahn, P.H. (ed.), *Children and nature: psychological, sociocultural and evolutionary investigations*. Cambridge, MA: MIT Press, pp. 305–327.

Rose, K.A., Morgan, I.G., Ip, J., Kifley, A., Huynh, S., Smith, W. and Mitchell, P. (2008) Outdoor activity reduces the prevalence of myopia in children, *Ophthalmology*, 115(8), pp. 1279–1285.

Sandseter, E.B.H. (2010) *Scaryfunny: a qualitative study of risky play among preschool children*. Trondheim: Norwegian University of Science and Technology.

Sandseter, E.B.H. and Kennair, L.E.O. (2011) Children's risky play from an evolutionary perspective: the anti-phobic effects of thrilling experiences. *Evolutionary Psychology*, 9(2), pp. 257–284.

Sandseter, E.B.H., Rasmus, K. and Sando, O.J. (2021) The prevalence of risky play in young children's indoor and outdoor free play. *Early Childhood Education Journal*, 49(2), pp. 303–312.

Sobel, D. (1993) *Children's special places*. Detroit. Wayne State University Press.

Song, R., Chen, Q., Zhang, Y., Jia, Q., He, H., Gao, T. and Qiu, L. (2022) Psychophysiological restorative potential in cancer patients by virtual reality (VR)-based perception of natural environment. *Frontiers in. Psychology*, 13(1003497), pp. 1–14. doi: 10.3389/fpsyg.2022.1003497.

Stewart, D. and Eccleston, J. (2020) *Scotland's People and Nature Survey 2019/20 – outdoor recreation, health, and environmental attitudes modules*. NatureScot Research Report No. 1227. Available at: https://www.nature.scot/sites/default/files/2020-10/NatureScot%20Research%20Report%20 1227%20-%20Scotland%27s%20People%20and%20Nature%20Survey%202019-20%20-%20 outdoor%20recreation%2C%20health%2C%20and%20environmental%20attitudes%20modules. pdf (Accessed 20.8.2024).

Stobbs, N. (2024) *Let's make Worcester a vibrant and playful city*. Available at: https://playworcester. co.uk/blog/f/lets-make-worcester-a-vibrant-and-playful-city-by-niki-stobbs (Accessed 17 January 2025).

Thal, L. (2014) Attention-deficit hyperactivity disorder and exposure to nature in college students. Available at: https://mospace.umsystem.edu/xmlui/handle/10355/44338 (Accessed 21 August 2024).

van den Berg, A.E. and van den Berg, C.G. (2011) A comparison of children with ADHD in a natural and built setting, *Child: Care, Health and Development*, 37(3), pp. 430–439. doi: 10.1111/j.1365-2214.2010.01172. x.

Waite, S. and Pratt, N. (2009) Theoretical perspectives on learning outside the classroom – relationships between learning and place, in Waite, S. (ed.) *Children learning outside the classroom*. London: Sage, pp. 24–38.

Wang, X., Rodiek, S., Wu, C., Chen, Y. and Li, Y. (2016) Stress recovery and restorative effects of viewing different urban park scenes in Shanghai, China, *Urban Forestry & Urban Greening*, 15, pp. 112–122. doi: https://doi.org/10.1016/j.ufug.2015.12.003.

Williams, D.R. and Vaske, J.J. (202) *The measurement of place attachment: validity and gereralizability of a psychometric approach*. A paper written and prepared by U.S. Department of Agriculture, Forest Services, Rocky Mountain Research Station, pp. 1–28.

7
A mindful approach

Introduction

We live in an increasingly fast paced and busy world, where we are often bombarded with sensory stimulation from all directions. Technology, and the relentless pace of modern life, means that there is always something clamouring for our attention, and our senses are being continually aroused. This sensory overload can often lead to stress, anxiety and difficulty in focusing. It is as if our minds must constantly race to keep up with the barrage of information and stimuli around us. For children, this can be even more overwhelming. Their developing brains are soaking up everything around them, but they do not yet have the ability to filter and process it all effectively. The result can be a sense of disorientation and heightened anxiety. In this context, mindfulness can help achieve calmness. By teaching children to pause, breathe and focus on the present moment, we can help them to navigate this sensory rich world with much more clarity. Mindfulness offers a sanctuary from chaos and sensory bombardment, allowing children to reconnect with their inner world, and find peace amongst the noise. They learn to tune in to their own inner world by balancing the external sensory inputs with moments of quiet reflection. This chapter explores the significant role that mindfulness can play in allowing individuals, and especially those who have experienced trauma, to experience calmness and focus beyond the stresses of the past or future. In this chapter we will consider what mindfulness is, how it can be used to support children and useful strategies for including mindfulness within our practice.

Mindfulness

Over the last several years, mindfulness has come to the fore in our society. There are now many self-help books on mindfulness and apps that help us practise it. However, mindfulness is often defined loosely; it is one of those words we may use frequently with only a vague idea of what it means. Mindfulness is distinct from meditation although the two concepts are related. Mindfulness is about being fully present in the current moment, aware of thoughts and feelings but without judgement and it can be practised in any activity such as eating or walking. Meditation is a more structured practise where you set time aside to focus inwards often using techniques like repeating a mantra, visualising or focusing on breath. Meditation can help cultivate mindfulness, but it is a specific activity rather than a general approach to life.

Creswell (2017) views mindfulness as a technique which involves paying full attention to your thoughts, feelings and bodily sensations. Kabat-Zinn (2001, p.4) goes further, defining mindfulness as a "form of consciousness that involves paying attention in a particular way: on purpose, in the present moment, and non-judgmentally". This definition positions mindfulness as something very intentional that requires action, awareness and an ability to put aside our judgement and assumptions. This is not easy, which is why mindfulness experts stress the importance of practising mindfulness regularly and finding those techniques that work for us as individuals.

As an approach that promotes calm and restores focus, practising mindfulness can be useful for people of all ages and backgrounds. Mindfulness is one of the most pervasive and fastest growing interventions in adult mental health (Prakash *et al.*, 2017) and is supported by a robust evidence base (Semple & Burke, 2019). More recently, however, there has been a focus on the effectiveness of mindfulness for children and young people (Saunders & Kober, 2020) and some research supports the use of mindfulness-based interventions in the treatment of anxiety for children as young as five (Ruiz-Íñiguez *et al.*, 2020). Mindfulness can be particularly helpful for children as it provides them with a skill that that they can use throughout their lives to support their wellbeing; it can play a significant role in supporting emotional regulation, improving focus and reducing anxiety (Zelazo & Lyons, 2012). Baudon & Jachens (2021) suggest that mindfulness is an intervention that can help children deal with the increasingly uncertain future and is particularly effective in supporting children who are anxious about war or climate catastrophe. When it comes to more generalised anxiety, mindfulness aims to bring attention back to the present moment and to minimise unhelpful rumination (Gomez *et al.*, 2017). Mindfulness has the benefit that it does not require special resources or input from another person. When a child has learned mindfulness techniques, they can implement these approaches at any time and in any environment, making this an empowering tool for children to support their own wellbeing. The next sections will explore in more detail the benefits of mindfulness for children.

Mindfulness and self-regulation

There is growing evidence that mindfulness can support a child's self-regulation in several important ways:

- Through practising mindful breathing and meditation children learn to calm their minds and their bodies. This can help reduce impulsivity and improve attention, allowing them to make more thoughtful decisions.
- Mindfulness can help a child differentiate between a thought and a feeling. It enables children to become more aware of their emotions, and to be able to recognise them as they arise. Such awareness is an important first step in managing emotions effectively.
- Mindfulness techniques have been shown to lower stress levels by teaching children to remain present in the moment, and not get overwhelmed by negative thoughts. Lower stress can result in better emotional control.
- By practising mindfulness children can develop better control over their impulses. They learn to pause and consider their responses rather than reacting immediately out of

anger or frustration. This more measured approach is crucial for self-regulation.
- Practising mindfulness can help children build resilience, providing them with tools to cope with challenges and setbacks. They become more adept at managing demanding situations without becoming overwhelmed.
- Mindfulness can encourage a reflective approach to problems. It allows children to take a step back from the situation and assess it calmly.

In a meta study of mindfulness research carried out post pandemic, Bockman and Yu (2023) found that the use of mindfulness techniques had mixed success in promoting emotional regulation with a general population of young children. However, when it came to children in need of additional support, the positive effects of mindfulness on self-regulation were significantly greater. This included children who had delays in development, as well as those who were struggling with self-regulation.

Mindfulness to counter anxiety

Fear and anxiety are commonly experienced by children and young people. For many children, these difficult emotions are experienced infrequently and are short-lived (Beesdo-Baum & Knappe, 2012). However, for a growing number of children, the symptoms develop into more profound anxiety disorders, characterised by excessive and persistent fears, avoidance of certain situations due to anticipation of threat, and an associated disruption in many aspects of the child's life (Creswell *et al.*, 2020). Odgers *et al.* (2020) argue strongly that mindfulness techniques are not sufficient alone to treat children's severe anxiety, and more intensive interventions delivered by a trained specialist will be necessary to support the child. Indeed, cognitive-behavioural-therapy- (CBT) based interventions are currently considered the best approaches for the prevention and treatment of childhood anxiety disorders (James *et al.*, 2015) and this will be considered in Chapter 8. However, mindfulness may be helpful in supporting children with transient anxiety or, indeed, as an intervention when helping a child who is waiting for specialist input. There is some evidence that mindfulness practices can help calm the limbic system (see Chapter 2). By engaging in mindfulness children can learn to self soothe and manage their anxiety levels. The practice vignette below explores how mindfulness can be used to support a child's emotional wellbeing in a crisis situation.

 Practice vignette

At Forest School, Mikey and Samir are building dens together. Their play continues cooperatively for some time as they construct a den against neighbouring trees. However, conflict arises when both children want a particular stick, which has an unusual curve to it. Mikey says he saw it first; however, Samir is adamant that it is his to use as he had picked it up and used it to construct a door to his den. The conflict escalates and Mikey kicks Samir's den causing it to partially collapse, then takes the stick to use in his own construction. Laura, the play worker, notices that Samir is very upset and intervenes gently. She notices that Mikey is still building his den; she will chat with him later but for now he is okay; however, Samir is inconsolable. He is sobbing loudly and now says urgently that he can't breathe. Indeed, he

A mindful approach 93

is looking increasingly terrified and is showing all the outward symptoms of a panic attack. Laura remains calm throughout. She takes deep breaths to maintain her own composure. She reminds him that he is safe and that she is there to help. Laura encourages Samir to take slow deep breaths. She breathes with him for several breaths. Then she encourages him to count his breaths, inhaling deeply through the nose for a count of four, holding for four and then exhaling through the mouth for a count of four. Laura keeps a watchful eye on Samir and notices that his breathing appears more controlled now. Laura asks Samir to focus on the sensation of the breath entering and leaving his body, together they place a hand on their stomach to feel it rise and fall. Now that Samir has more control, Laura helps him focus on his senses. Together they do the 5,4,3,2,1 exercise, identifying five things that Samir can see, four things he can make and touch, three things he can hear, two things he can smell and one thing he can taste. Laura continues to reassure Samir and remind him that he is okay. She uses phrases like "this feeling will go away soon" or "you're safe right now". Once the panic has subsided, she talks with Samir about what he experienced and what helped him to calm down. This can provide valuable insights and help him feel understood.

After the incident Laura reflects on the situation. She decides to make practising mindfulness a regular part of the sessions so that children have skills to use in moments of intense anxiety. After the session she talks with Samir's dad who tells her that this has happened on previous occasions. Laura gives Sam's dad some mindfulness resources but also suggests talking it over with their GP.

Critical question

What are the potential benefits of teaching mindfulness techniques to all children?

Basic mindfulness techniques

Adults can support children to become mindful through a variety of different techniques and approaches. The main ones are outlined below:

- **Breathing exercises** – examples of these are counted breath and box breathing. Box breathing is a mindful relaxation technique which involves focusing on a square object and following a four-sided breathing pattern (inhale, hold, exhale, hold). This technique can be particularly helpful in easing panic and controlling hyperventilation (Ahmed *et al.*, 2021)
- **5,4,3,2,1 sensory approach** – this involves identifying five things you can see, four things you can touch, three things you can hear, two things you can smell, and one thing you can taste. This method was developed by Betty Erikson (2038-2019) and is quoted in Quick (2013)
- **Mindful consumption of food** – this is where the individual is encouraged to spend time focusing on a food item, taking account of its texture, taste and/or smell before eating it (Hong, 2018).
- **Body scan** – this practice focuses on developing an awareness of current physical sensations. Attention is moved systematically through the body in sequence, usually from

head to toes. The aim of the exercise is to direct non-judgemental attention to each part of the body rather than to deliberately promote relaxation (Thompson & Gauntlett-Gilbert, 2008) although many people do find this process relaxing.
- **Visualisation** – this involves guiding children. The objective is to create calming mental images that help soothe and focus their minds. The serene images help children to manage stress and anxiety offering a mental retreat and tranquillity. By regularly practising such visualisations children can develop a valuable tool to support their emotional wellbeing.

Critical questions

- How might cultural differences and family backgrounds influence children's receptiveness/engagement with mindfulness practices?
- How can practitioners ensure that mindfulness practices are inclusive and accessible to all children?
- Are there any ethical considerations surrounding the implementation of mindfulness practices with children, particularly in terms of consent?
- How much do mindfulness practices impact children's social interactions and relationships with peers and adults?

Some mindfulness activities

The following mindful activities provide an excellent introduction to using mindfulness with children. These activities do not require many resources and can be adapted for different ages and abilities.

A mindful walk

The objective of this activity is to help children practise mindfulness by focusing on their senses during a walk in their local environment. Explain to the children that they will be going on a special walk where they will pay close attention to everything around them. Encourage the children to walk slowly and quietly notice as much as they can with their senses. Begin by taking a few deep breaths together to centre and ground everyone. Ask the children to focus on their breath as they start walking, noticing how their feet feel as they touch the ground. They can experiment with walking lightly or heavily, small steps or large steps, fast or slowly. Ask the children to look around and notice colours, shapes and patterns. Encourage them to take in the details of the leaves, flowers, trees and any other natural elements around them. Next have the children listen closely to the sounds around them. This could be birds chirping, leaves rustling or distant traffic. Encourage the children to identify as many sounds as they can. Tell the children to take deep breaths and notice any smells in the air. This might include the scent of flowers, grass, earth after rain or other environmental aromas. Ask the children to gently touch natural objects such as stones, leaves, tree bark and describe how they feel. Are they rough, smooth, warm or cold?

After the walk find a quiet place to sit together and encourage the children to share their experiences. What did they notice? How did they feel during the walk? The children can write about or draw their favourite part of the walk. Finish with a few more deep breaths together. Remind the children that they can practise mindfulness anytime, anywhere, by simply paying attention to their surroundings and their senses. This activity helps children slow down, engage with their environment and develop a greater sense of presence and calm.

Rainbow relaxation

Get the children to lie in a comfortable position and focus on breaths. You are now going to lead them through a visualisation based on a rainbow.

Imagine you are lying in a beautiful meadow. Feel the grass beneath you and the breeze on your face. There is a wonderful smell of flowers and fresh grass. Ask the children to imagine a blue sky with a beautiful rainbow. Then tell them to focus on the colours of the rainbow starting with red. Encourage the children to focus on each colour and to think of something that makes them happy or calm in that colour.

Clay sculpting

This activity encourages sensory awareness and creativity. Provide each child with a piece of modelling clay. Encourage them to mould a shape from the clay, paying close attention to the texture and how it feels in their hands. Suggest they create something that represents a peaceful place or a peaceful object. Talk together about the artwork that each child has created.

Emotion doodling

This helps children express and understand their emotions through art and creativity. Ask the children to think about how they are feeling. Encourage them to draw or doodle their emotions on paper using colours, shapes and images that represent their feelings. Afterwards, discuss their drawings and what emotions they chose to express.

Mindful breathing together

Help children to focus on their breath and build connections. Pair the children up and have them sit back-to-back with their friend. Ask them to synchronise their breathing, feeling the rise and fall of their partner's breath against their back. Encourage them to focus on the rhythm of their combined breaths and how it feels to be connected.

Mindful eating

This is a particularly useful activity which enables children to focus mindfully on their senses. Get everyone sitting quietly and focusing on their breathing. Give each child a raisin. First, ask the children look at the raisin. Next, tell them to smell the raisin. Then get them to place the raisin on their tongue but tell them not to chew it. Finally, have them bite into the raisin and eat it focusing on the taste. This activity can be extended by thinking about the raisin as a grape, of the people who picked it, packaged it and transported it and practising gratitude.

> **REFLECTIVE TASK**
>
> Plan and use at least one of the activities above with a child or group of children. Reflect on the activity using the prompts in Table 7.1.

Table 7.1 Reflection on a mindfulness activity

Describe the activity
How did it go?
What were the benefits you observed?
Were there any challenges?
What might you do differently next time?
What have you learned?

Exploring the mind-body connection

Emotions are embodied. In other words, emotions are not just abstract feelings in our mind but are also experienced physically in our bodies. Examples of this include how your heart races when you're scared, how your stomach feels queasy when you're anxious or how muscles tense up when a person is angry. These physical sensations are the body's way of expressing and experiencing emotions. By understanding how our emotions manifest in our bodies we can better understand and manage our emotional experiences. This idea is fundamental in practices that focus on somatic experiences. Some examples are explored below.

Yoga

Yoga is an ancient practice that was developed in India. It involves meditation, movement and a focus on breathing. In the last decade there has been a growth in interest in yoga for children. Some schools offer yoga sessions, and there are many clubs and classes available in communities. Proponents of yoga for children argue that it can have a range of benefits for them, including physical benefits (such as improving balance, strength, endurance, aerobic capacity and flexibility), body awareness, self-efficacy (as children work to perfect the movements) and academic prowess (specifically focus and concentration). However, yoga has even more benefits for mental health and self-esteem (Nanthakumar, 2018). In a meta study Kerekes *et al.* (2023) argued that existing studies have demonstrated promising results regarding yoga in enhancing children's mental health, stress management and self-esteem. Moreover, most children who participated in yoga sessions found them fun and enjoyable.

However, there are several criticisms and caveats in relation to children's yoga. First, it is important to remember that children's bodies are still developing, and it is crucial that a trained person delivers the yoga sessions to avoid physical injury. A trained practitioner will know what exercises are appropriate for a particular age and be able to adapt their approach accordingly. Some families may have religious or cultural objections to their children participating in yoga sessions because of the links to Eastern philosophies. Yoga may not be inclusive to children with physical disabilities.

Progressive muscle relaxation

Progressive muscle relaxation (PMR) is a technique used to reduce anxiety and stress. By systematically tensing and relaxing different muscle groups in the body, this provides a useful way for children to learn how to manage tension and find a state of calm. Focusing on how tension and relaxation feel within the body, PMR encourages a deeper awareness of bodily sensations. However, PMR has been criticised because it is whilst it can help to relax muscles, the underlying emotional symptoms might persist. As such PMR can provide temporary relief from muscle tension and stress, but may not offer a long-term solution for chronic stress or anxiety,

Case study: Kimberley Pena, an embodied approach

The following case study is provided by Kimberly Pena, a dance psychotherapist who works in the NHS. Kim is passionate about movement to promote wellbeing and healing, particularly for individuals who have struggled with body image. Here, Kim reflects upon her own practice, drawing upon dance psychotherapy theory and examples from her work.

> In a world where we are often cognitively overwhelmed and existing in bodies that feel burdened, often frozen by the weight of our troubles, focusing on the body through embodied ways of understanding can be helpful. Dance movement psychotherapy can be found in mental health settings, both within the NHS and private practice. Supporting psychological, physical and social health through the moving body is not new, but a developmentally innate process we have neglected. Our earliest ways of understanding and making sense of ourselves and the world around us was through movement and touch. We naturally prioritised somatic processing (focusing on healing where our trauma is held in the body) before our thinking brains took the driving seat.
>
> Whether we are trained 'embodied practitioner'" or not, we can all relate to that deep, visceral 'gut feeling' that often counteracts our rational thoughts and ideas about a particular decision/person/experience. We have mostly tuned out of this 'felt sense' but it is what embodied practices, such as dance movement psychotherapy invites us to return to. Through somatic awareness and embodiment, we recognise that our body is a holding space for a 'felt level' of pre-verbal understanding (Gendlin, 1996).
>
> From its beginnings in the 1940s to its accreditation as a post-graduate qualification in the 1980s, dance movement psychotherapy has amassed a robust evidence base that has strengthened the case for its role in healthcare, for example, when supporting people recovering from an eating disorder. Offering dance movement psychotherapy to this client group creates space for the client to rebuild and reclaim their relationship with their body.
>
> A participant from a dance movement psychotherapy group for eating disorders (EDs) reflected:
>> I was extremely nervous going into the first session, but I soon felt supported to and listened to. It was really eye opening to hear other people's experiences of their ED; it

allowed me to appreciate parts of my body and helped me find reasons to like myself more, and it also helped improve my body image. I was inspired to see and hear from other people around the same age as I was express how they felt about their struggles, and it made me feel less isolated and alienated. I found most of it extremely helpful, but the 'check ins' were the most helpful, where we would take time to connect with how we were and then reflect on how things were with our illness. This helped me reconnect to myself beyond my identity associated with my eating disorder.

Outside of the session room the profession of dance movement psychotherapy has much to offer other colleagues working with young people and families. One of these areas is how we tend to our own moving, thinking, feeling body when we are supporting more vulnerable individuals to be seen, heard and understood. We are often invited to practise mindfulness as part of self-care so that our own wellbeing is sustained as we carry out these frequently intensive roles. I urge the reader to also consider using 'bodyfulness' - a practice that goes beyond passive awareness and into action, entering a state of active awareness, meaning- making and letting go, with and through the moving body in a creative and playful way.

Creative movement invites us to return to previous experiences held emotionally and physically in our bodies, honour them and then re-tread the path to our authentic self without the need for words or sense-making. In this process unfiltered feelings are allowed to flow, creating an internal dialogue between body and mind to reclaim one's rhythm of life.

Critical questions

- Kim speaks of being in a state where we are often "cognitively overwhelmed and existing in bodies that feel burdened". Do you agree? What do you think are some of the factors that cause us to feel this way?
- Kim reminds us that "our earliest means of understanding and making sense of ourselves and the world around us was through movement and touch". This suggests that children may be able to tune into their bodies more naturally than adults. What examples can you find from practice to support this idea? At what point does this change for children and why?
- What does Kim mean by "bodyfulness"? How can we use this concept to support our work with children and families?
- How could you incorporate dance into your own practice to support children's wellbeing?

Conclusion

It is little wonder that there is so much interest in mindfulness for children. The benefits for adults have long been known and there are many evidence-based interventions, particularly related to anxiety and stress management. However, as we experience increasing levels of anxiety and poor mental health among children and young people, there is a growing recognition that mindfulness may provide a useful approach for practitioners to support children's wellbeing. In a time when financial resources are tight, mindfulness is particularly attractive as it does not demand any specialist equipment, and anyone can be trained to do it. Moreover, is it being an approach that children can be taught to self-administer, giving them ownership and responsibility for their own wellbeing, which in turn fosters self-efficacy. It is not, however, a panacea. Where children have experienced multiple adversity or profound trauma, mindfulness alone is unlikely to provide a solution when used in isolation. The next chapter will consider talking therapies and cognitive approaches, which provide further tools that practitioners can use to support the children and families they work with.

A mindful approach: key points

- Mindfulness is a practice that enables children to focus on the present moment, without judgement. As such it helps children to become more aware of their thoughts, feelings and bodily sensations.
- Mindfulness has been associated with several benefits for children including improved sleep, better focus, stress and anxiety reduction, calmness and relaxation.
- Being introduced to mindfulness can provide children and young people with a tool that they can use to help them self-regulate.
- There is a powerful interplay between thoughts, emotions and physical health. Body-based (somatic) interventions can play a key role in promoting wellbeing.

ADDITIONAL RESOURCES

- Young Minds website https://www.youngminds.org.uk

This website has a range of information, resources and signposts regarding children's mental health and emotional wellbeing.

- BBC bitesize https://www.bbc.co.uk/bitesize/articles/zhmtg2p

This website has several helpful resources for parents about mindfulness and how to incorporate it into a child's routines and daily activities.

- Dr Wayne Johnson's Technology, Entertainment and Design (TED) talk on mindfulness with children mhttps://www.ted.com/talks/dr_wayne_johnson_mindfulness_the_solution_for_anxious_kids?subtitle=en

Dr Johnson makes a compelling case for the benefits of mindfulness for children's mental health and wellbeing.

- The Association for Dance Movement Psychotherapy UK website https://admp.org.uk

This website has useful information about dance psychotherapy.

References

Ahmed, A., Gayatri Devi, R. and Jothi Priya, A. (2021) Effect of Box Breathing Technique on Lung Function Test. *Journal of Pharmaceutical Medicine*, 33(58A), pp. 25-31.

Baudon, P. and Jachens, L. (2021) A scoping review of interventions for the treatment of eco-anxiety. *International Journal of Environmental Research and Public Health*, 18(18), p. 9636.

Beesdo-Baum, K. and Knappe, S. (2012) Developmental epidemiology of anxiety disorders. *Child and Adolescent Psychiatric Clinics*, 21(3), pp. 457-478.

Beesdo-Baum, K., Lieb, R. and Wittchen, H.-U. (2013) Anxiety disorders as early stages of malignant psychopathological long-term outcomes: results of the 10-years prospective EDSP Study, *Comprehensive Psychiatry*, 54(8), e16. doi: https://doi.org/10.1016/j.comppsych.2013.07.006.

Bockmann, J.O. and Yu, S.Y. (2023) Using mindfulness-based interventions to support self-regulation in young children: a review of the literature. *Early Childhood Education Journal*, 51(4), pp. 693-703.

Creswell, C., Waite, P. and Hudson, J. (2020) Practitioner review: anxiety disorders in children and young people – assessment and treatment. *Journal of Child Psychology and Psychiatry*, 61(6), pp. 628-643.

Creswell, J.D. (2017) Mindfulness interventions. *Annual Review of Psychology*, 68, pp. 491-516.

Damasio, A.R. (1999) *The feelings of what happens*. London: William Heinemann.

Ellis, H. (1923) *The dance of life*. Cambridge: Houghton Mifflin Co.

Gendlin, E.T. (1996) *Focusing-oriented psychotherapy: a manual of the experiential method*. New York: Guilford Press.

Gomez, J., Hoffman, H.G., Bistricky, S.L., Gonzalez, M., Rosenberg, L., Sampaio, M., Garcia-Palacios, A., Navarro-Haro, M.V., Alhalabi, W., Rosenberg, M. and Meyer III, W.J. (2017) The use of virtual reality facilitates dialectical behavior therapy® "observing sounds and visuals" mindfulness skills training exercises for a Latino patient with severe burns: a case study. *Frontiers in Psychology*, 8, p. 1611.

Hofmann, S.G. and Gómez, A.F. (2017) Mindfulness-based interventions for anxiety and depression, *Psychiatric Clinics*, 40(4), pp. 739-749.

Hong, P.Y., Hanson, M.D., Lishner, D.A., Kelso, S.L. and Steinert, S.W. (2018) A field experiment examining mindfulness on eating enjoyment and behaviour in children, *Mindfulness*, 9(10), pp. 1748-1756.

James, A.C., James, G., Cowdrey, F.A., Soler, A. and Choke, A. (2015) Cognitive behavioural therapy for anxiety disorders in children and adolescents, *Cochrane Database of Systematic Reviews*, 2. doi: https://doi.org/10.1002/14651858.cd004690.pub4.

Kabat-Zinn, J. (2001) *Mindfulness meditation for everyday life*. London: Piatkus.

Kerekes, N., Söderström, A., Holmberg, C. and Ahlström, B.H. (2024) Yoga for children and adolescents: a decade-long integrative review on feasibility and efficacy in school-based and psychiatric care interventions. *Journal of Psychiatric Research*, 180, pp. 489-499.

Khunti, K., Boniface, S., Norris, E., De Oliveira, C.M. and Shelton, N. (2023) The effects of yoga on mental health in school-aged children: a systematic review and narrative synthesis of randomised control trials, *Clinical Child Psychology and Psychiatry*, 28(3), pp. 1217-1238. doi: https://doi.org/10.1177/13591045221136016.

Meekums, B. (2007) Dance movement therapy in Britain: pioneers of a profession. Available at: academia.edu weblinkhttps://scholar.google.co.uk/scholar?hl=en&as_sdt=0%2C5&as_vis=1&q=Meekums%2C+%282007%29+Dance+movement+therapy+in+Britain%3A+Pioneers+of+a+profession&btnG=

Nanthakumar, C. (2018) The benefits of yoga in children, *Journal of Integrative Medicine*, 16(1), pp. 14-19.

Odgers, K., Dargue, N., Creswell, C., Jones, M.P. and Hudson, J.L. (2020) The limited effect of mindfulness-based interventions on anxiety in children and adolescents: a meta-analysis, *Clinical Child and Family Psychology Review*, 23(3), pp. 407-426.

Prakash, R.S., Whitmoyer, P., Aldao, A. and Schirda, B. (2017) Mindfulness and emotion regulation in older and young adults, *Aging & Mental Health*, 21(1), pp. 77-87.

Quick, E.K. (2013) *Solution focused anxiety management: a treatment and training manual*. San Diego, CA: Academic Press Inc.

Ruiz-Íñiguez, R., Santed German, M.A., Burgos-Julián, F.A., Díaz-Silveira, C. and Carralero Montero, A. (2020) Effectiveness of mindfulness-based interventions on anxiety for children and adolescents: a systematic review and meta-analysis, *Early Intervention in Psychiatry*, 14(3), pp. 263-274.

Sandel, S., Chaiklin, S. and Ohn, A. (eds.) (1993) *Foundations of dance/movement therapy: the life and work of Marian Chace*. Columbia, MD: Marian Chace Memorial Fund.

Saunders, D. and Kober, H. (2020) Mindfulness-based intervention development for children and adolescents, *Mindfulness*, 11(8), pp. 1868–1883.

Semple, R.J. and Burke, C. (2019) State of the research: physical and mental health benefits of mindfulness-based interventions for children and adolescents. *OBM Integrative and Complementary Medicine*, 4(1), pp. 1–58.

Sheets-Johnstone, M. (2010) Why is movement therapeutic? Keynote address, 44th American Dance Therapy Association Conference, October 9, 2009, Portland, OR. *American Journal of Dance Therapy*, 32, pp. 2–15.

Thompson, M. and Gauntlett-Gilbert, J. (2008) Mindfulness with children and adolescents: effective clinical application, *Clinical Child Psychology and Psychiatry*, 13(3), pp. 395–407.

Zelazo, P.D. and Lyons, K.E. (2012) The potential benefits of mindfulness training in early childhood: a developmental social cognitive neuroscience perspective, *Child Development Perspectives*, 6(2), pp. 154–160.

8
Talking therapies

Introduction

The NHS defines talking therapies as "psychological treatments for mental and emotional problems" (NHS, 2024). There are many kinds of talking therapy, but what they all have in common is that they involve talking with a trained therapist. Delivering talking therapy interventions requires extensive professional training and registration with a regulating body. Hence, these are not approaches that can be delivered by non-specialist practitioners without them undergoing additional training. However, this chapter provides an overview of some of the main talking therapies and explores a few activities that practitioners can use to support children and families when they are awaiting professional treatment. In the chapter, we explore the benefits of cognitive approaches such as cognitive behavioural therapy (CBT), dialectical behaviour therapy (DBT) and acceptance and commitment therapy (ACT). We explore practice vignettes that show these therapies in action. The case study for this chapter is a conversation with Eirian and Natasha, practitioners who use talking therapies as part of their work to support children and young people who are care-experienced.

An overview of talking therapies

We all know how beneficial it can be to talk through our problems with a trusted individual in our lives. Talking can help us problem solve, make us feel that we are not alone and help us feel heard and understood. Talking therapies take this one step further as they involve talking with a trained therapist with the objective of addressing emotional and psychological issues that we may be experiencing. There are many distinct types of talking therapy some of which are about exploring our innermost thoughts and feelings, whilst others more pragmatically focus on problem solving. Psychodynamic therapy (based on the work of Sigmund Freud) involves exploring the unconscious mind and how it influences thoughts, feelings and behaviours. Jungian psychotherapy seeks to bring together conscious and unconscious elements in a holistic approach that prioritises self-understanding and personal growth.

Counselling

Counselling is a form of professional guidance where a councillor helps individuals explore and address their personal and emotional issues. In counselling sessions, children can talk

DOI: 10.4324/9781003459668-10

freely about things that are upsetting them. This can help them understand their emotions more fully and can provide a listening and non-judgemental space for the child to feel heard. School counsellors can be a particularly helpful resource for young people as they are easy to access and the counselling is delivered in a context that is familiar to the child.

Family group conferencing (FGC)

Family group conferencing (FGC) is a family-led, decision-making process where the extended family and friends network come together to create a plan for a child's welfare. This process is facilitated by an independent coordinator who helps the family prepare for the meeting. The child is often involved in the conferencing, often with their own advocate.

Cognitive approaches

Cognitive approaches focus on how our thoughts influence our feelings and behaviour. In understanding and changing thought processes, individuals can experience enhanced emotional and psychological wellbeing. When considering the use of talking therapies with children and young people, there are many considerations. Children need to be of an age and ability where they can participate fully in such approaches and benefit from them. Hence these approaches are not suitable for very young or non-verbal children. Approaches need to be tailored to the developmental needs, personality and preferences of the child. If a child has experienced severe trauma, talking about it too soon can re-traumatise them. Building trust will be essential for such children, who may have been let down or exploited in the past. Similarly, if a child is currently in a crisis situation, immediate calming and stabilisation would be the priority and one would not want to use talking therapies until the time was right (this is discussed further in the case study later in the chapter). Moreover, talking therapies rely on the child's engagement and desire to participate. Resistance from the child will result in the intervention being ineffective. Consequently from the outset, building a strong and trustful relationship is crucial prior to entering into any kind of therapy.

Creating a therapeutic relationship

Prior to any intervention, it is important that a strong and trustful relationship is created. The importance of relationship building cannot be overstated and there is evidence to suggest that the quality of the therapeutic relationship is even more important than the actual intervention in predicting how successful treatment is likely to be (Kidd *et al.*, 2017). The aspects of practice that make up this relationship are often referred to as *common factors*; this refers to elements that are present across different therapeutic approaches and contribute to their effectiveness. Common factors might include:

- The quality of the relationship between the therapist and the individual receiving therapy. A strong, trusting and collaborative bond is crucial for effective therapy (Leahy, 2008).
- The therapist's ability to empathise with the feelings being shared, which in turn helps the individual to feel heard, validated and supported.
- The therapist's competence (skills, knowledge and ability to guide the intervention) which instils confidence and trust that the person being treated is in safe hands.

So far, these common factors derive from the therapist. However, there are also common factors that are intrinsic to the individual receiving treatment, including:

- Motivation, readiness and willingness to engage in the therapeutic process. This is because people with higher motivation are more likely to work towards goals and undertake home-based tasks.
- The belief that the therapy can work and hope for a good outcome.

Ideally these common factors underpin the intervention that is to be provided and make it more likely that the intervention will have a positive outcome. Whilst these factors are important in talking therapies, they are relevant to all other modalities of intervention. Fostering these factors within our work with children and young people can provide a solid foundation for all the approaches we might use to support them (Prowle & Hodgkins, 2020).

Cognitive behavioural therapy (CBT)

Cognitive behavioural therapy (CBT) is based on the concept that your physical feelings, thoughts and behaviours are interlinked in a negative cycle which can perpetuate emotional difficulties (Greimel et al., 2011). CBT approaches can provide the individual with techniques for managing difficult emotions such as fear or anger (Clark, 2013), and a large body of research has shown that CBT is effective in treating childhood anxiety disorders (James et al., 2020). There are a variety of CBT techniques that parents and educators can introduce when working with children who suffer from anxiety. Such anxiety may include:

- Unhelpful patterns of thought
- Generalised anxiety
- Social anxiety
- Compulsive thoughts
- Specific phobias
- Catastrophic interpretations
- Suicidal ideation.

A CBT intervention is preceded by a robust assessment which includes an exploration of the issues being experienced, home conditions and support networks and a risk assessment. The intervention usually takes place over six weekly sessions which can be delivered in a face-to-face context, over the telephone or online.

CBT is a 'here and now' therapy (Sakdalan et al., 2010) which focuses on the present moment, rather than delving into the past. The foundation of CBT is an understanding of the CBT triangle in which thoughts, feelings and behaviours are interrelated and go round in a cycle. So, for example, if a child is depressed, they might feel sluggish, tired and unmotivated, this would affect their negative thoughts about going out ("I can't be bothered", "I am not up to it today"). This, in turn, may lead to behaviours such as withdrawal or avoidance, which then intensify the original feelings resulting in a self-perpetuating cycle. This is shown in Figure 8.1.

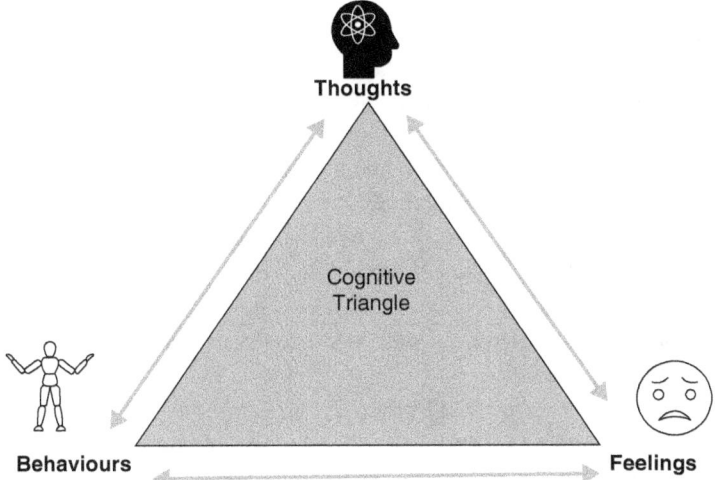

Figure 8.1 CBT triangle

There are several techniques which may be used in a CBT intervention. These include.

- **Cognitive restructuring:** This is a technique that has been successfully used to help people change the way they think. The goal is to replace unhelpful thoughts (cognitive distortions) with more balanced thoughts. A good example of this might be a child who believes that nobody wants to be their friend. By examining the evidence and finding examples of when peers were kind to them, they are able to challenge the unhelpful thought.
- **Behavioural ativation:** This is helpful when people are avoiding activities or not doing much as a result of their depression or anxiety. The aim is to re-build a balance of activities, to include routine activities (like brushing their teeth), necessary activities (such as completing homework) and pleasurable activities (things they enjoy or that help them to relax). By gradually creating a more balanced approach, a person will get a boost from completing activities, which then enhances self-efficacy.
- **Worry management:** This involves finding ways to manage worries. Where worries are real and you have control over them (for example, a child has an exam coming up), problem solving will help the child take practical steps to lessen the worry (such as creating a revision timetable or getting help with something they do not understand). Where worries are more hypothetical (for example, worries about the future, war or a hypothetical illness) postponement of worries to a designated time put aside for worrying can be very helpful.
- **Exposure and habituation:** This is helpful for specific fears. This approach entails exposing yourself to situations you find stressful by putting yourself in the situation (exposure) and then gradually allowing your mind and body to get used to it (habituation) and build up tolerance levels.

Some of these techniques are explored in the practice vignette below.

Practice vignette

Tammy is 15 years old and has always struggled with social anxiety. This has become much worse since COVID-19. Her attendance at school is very sporadic and she often leaves halfway through the day when she does attend. When she goes out, she often brings her mum for support and when alone she wears headphones and plain clothing to avoid drawing attention to herself. She reports feeling sick and shaky in social situations and often becomes anxious about blushing. She worries other people are judging her or that she will say something stupid. Her grades have dropped at school and teachers have said that she has become more withdrawn. She has stopped going out with her friends and playing for the local football team, which she loved previously.

Tammy has been referred to a CBT practitioner, Faiqa, for some support. They begin by exploring the CBT cycle and how this might look for someone with social anxiety. This helps Tammy understand the links between her thoughts, feelings and behaviours. For example, Faiqa explains that the anxious thoughts are likely to make the blushing more pronounced, which then makes Tammy worry even more about the blushing and whether other people have noticed. As home practice, Faiqa encourages Tammy to keep a thought diary to document the anxious thoughts before, during and after situations. This allows them to identify any patterns and triggers for Tammy's anxiety. They notice that Tammy is experiencing a lot of self-critical thoughts such as 'I'm embarrassing myself' or 'people think I'm stupid.' Faiqa introduces a technique called cognitive restructuring (challenging thoughts as they arise). Faiqa tells Tammy that this is like taking thoughts to trial, whereby both the evidence for and against the thought is considered. This enables Tammy to recognise that many of her thoughts are biased and helps her to come to more balanced conclusions. This builds Tammy's confidence, but she is still unconvinced that she is not embarrassing herself in social situations.

Faiqa suggests that an activity called behavioural experiments might help with this. Behavioural experiments requires you to expose yourself to uncomfortable situations and then monitor the outcome. Tammy decides to design a behavioural experiment whereby she asks a cashier in the shop where an item is. Before the experiment Tammy predicted that the cashier would be annoyed or dismissive. However, the cashier was very friendly and pointed her in the right direction. This gives her the confidence to try other situations such as going to the cinema with a close friend and ordering popcorn. By the final session of six, Tammy tells Faiqa that she was feeling anxious about certain social situations but she now felt that she had the techniques she needed to address anxiety when it arose.

Tammy expresses concern about slipping backwards after the sessions end. Faiqa reassures her that is quite normal and that there are things she can do to prevent relapsing, such as holding regular check-ins with herself to reflect on how she is feeling and how her anxiety has been of late. Faiqa also encourages Tammy to continue talking to those around her and practising the techniques she has learned. Tammy is now feeling nervous but optimistic about the future.

Critical questions

- What techniques does Faiqa use to support Tammy?
- Faiqa encourages Tammy to continue practising the techniques she has learned – why is this important?

Using CBT approaches in your practice

Whilst it is important that CBT interventions are led by a trained practitioner, there are many approaches that can be self-administered or that a non-specialist practitioner can use in practice to support children. This is especially important when waiting lists for professional services and CBT interventions are lengthy. These approaches can be carefully used to provide some help and symptom relief in the here and now. Mental health first aid training is available from many employers, who are recognising the importance of staff being able to provide initial support and signposting. "5 steps to mental wellbeing" (NHS, n.d.) outlines five things an individual can do to support their mental health and wellbeing, enabling them to feel more positive and able to get the most out of life. These five ways include mindfulness, physical activity, social connection, giving to others and learning new things.

However, there are also a variety of CBT techniques that parents and practitioners can introduce when working with children who are suffering from anxiety. These can be highly effective and can give children and young people important tools to manage anxiety.

- **Worry time:** Set aside a discrete period of time each day to focus entirely on worries and try to identify solutions. Children should then be encouraged to refocus attention during the day and save worrying until 'worry time' (Dippel *et al.*, 2024).
- **Psychoeducation:** This is a core element of CBT (Dolan *et al.*, 2021). The aim is to inform the child about common symptoms of anxiety and the function of this anxiety. Having this knowledge can help to normalise the experience of anxiety and help the child or young person feel empowered and work towards developing positive coping strategies.
- **Worry box:** A worry box is a container in which a child can safely store their worries. They can write or draw their anxious thoughts and place them in the box. This encourages the child to let go of the worry and focus on the present moment (Creswell *et al.*, 2020).

Dialectical behaviour therapy (DBT)

Dialectical behaviour therapy (DBT) is a form of CBT originally developed by Marsha Linehan (Linehan, 2014) to treat borderline personality disorder in adults. Over time, DBT has been adapted for use with children and adolescents, focusing on helping them develop skills to manage emotions, improve relationships and enhance overall wellbeing. DBT for children combines traditional CBT techniques with mindfulness practices and principles of acceptance.

One of the core components of DBT for children is the development of emotional regulation skills. It is important that children learn to identify and label their emotions, understand the triggers and consequences of their emotional responses and use strategies to moderate intense emotions. This process helps them gain better control over their emotional experiences and reduces emotional outbursts and dysregulation.

Another essential element of DBT is distress tolerance. Children are taught techniques to cope with distressing situations without resorting to maladaptive behaviours. The idea is to be able to sit with difficult emotions without trying to change them. These techniques include distraction, self-soothing and radical acceptance (acknowledging and accepting the full range of emotions), enabling children to tolerate difficult emotions and situations without feeling overwhelmed. Similarly, mindfulness is a foundational aspect of DBT. Children are encouraged to practise mindfulness to develop greater awareness of their thoughts, feelings and bodily sensations. Mindfulness exercises help them stay grounded in the present moment, reducing anxiety and enhancing their ability to respond to situations with clarity and calmness (see Chapter 7 for more on this).

Interpersonal effectiveness skills are also a significant part of DBT for children. These skills help children navigate social interactions more effectively, improving their ability to communicate their needs, set boundaries and resolve conflicts. By enhancing their interpersonal skills, children can build and maintain healthier relationships with peers, family members and teachers.

Behavioural strategies are used to reinforce positive behaviours and shape new behaviours in DBT for children. These strategies help children replace maladaptive behaviours with more constructive ones, fostering a sense of competence and achievement. Parent and caregiver involvement is an important aspect of DBT for children. Parents and caregivers are often included in the therapy process to reinforce the skills learned in sessions and provide consistent support at home. Training for parents might include learning DBT skills themselves, helping them to understand their child's emotional and behavioural challenges, and providing strategies to support their child's development. Hence DBT can be very holistic and multi-faceted, drawing together different techniques and approaches to meet the child's needs across different settings. This is explored in the practice vignette below.

 Practice vignette

Mateo is 11 years old and is experiencing difficulties with relationships at home, in school and at his football club. He finds it difficult to regulate his feelings which often overwhelm him. He finds anger particularly challenging and says he feels like a volcano. Using DBT approaches his therapist puts together a multi-faceted support programme. He teaches Mateo a range of mindfulness and breathing techniques to enable Mateo to become more grounded in the moment and more aware of his emotions and his body. The therapist helps Mateo to recognise and name different emotions. Together they make an emotion wheel to visualise his emotions. They discuss things he can do to manage difficult emotions, such as using his interest in drawing to calm down or kicking a football outside to diffuse situations at home. They discuss the importance of not reacting immediately, but taking a breath and proceeding mindfully, making a positive choice. Together they action plan for better interpersonal skills using the DEARMAN technique (Linehan, 2014):

Describe the situation
Express – explain your feelings
Assert – state your needs
Reinforce – explain the positive outcomes
Mindful – stay focused
Appear confident – use a confident tone and posture
Negotiate – be willing to compromise.

Mateo's mum and the teaching assistant in his class receive some brief training on DBT so that they can support Mateo and ensure a consistent approach. His football coach also receives a handout of the techniques Mateo has been practising. Mateo continues to practise the skills and slowly finds that he is much calmer and is having less frequent outbursts. The class teacher is so impressed by his progress that she shares the DEARMAN approach with the rest of the class.

Critical question

- How useful is the DEARMAN model for supporting children's self-regulation and interactions with others?

Acceptance and commitment therapy (ACT)

Acceptance and commitment therapy (ACT) is a form of psychotherapy that emphasises psychological flexibility and mindfulness. Originally developed for adults, ACT has been adapted to be effective for children and young people. The core principles of ACT, which are acceptance, mindfulness, cognitive defusion (loosening the grip of identity to provide more flexible ways of thinking) and values-based action, help children develop skills to manage their thoughts and emotions, cope with stress and engage in meaningful activities. In ACT, children are taught to observe their thoughts and feelings without judgement, allowing them to respond to challenges in a more adaptive way. This approach helps them build resilience and improve their overall wellbeing. By focusing on their personal values, children learn to make choices that align with what is important to them, fostering a sense of purpose and direction.

Overall, ACT provides children with practical tools to navigate life's difficulties, promoting emotional awareness, self-compassion and psychological flexibility. It is a valuable approach for helping children develop the skills they need to thrive in a complex and ever-changing world.

 Practice vignette

Nine-year-old Mia is suffering from anxiety, shame and anger after her father was sent to prison for theft. This practice vignette shows how ACT was used to help her manage her emotions and find ways to enjoy her life.

- **Acceptance:** The therapist helps Mia understand that it's okay to feel sad, angry or confused. Mia's feelings are validated, and she realises that her reactions are normal
- **Cognitive defusion:** The the therapist teaches Mia to see her thoughts as just tthoughts, not facts. For example, when Mia thinks her friends do not trust her not to steal, it is just a thought, not the reality.
- **Being present:** Mia learns mindfulness techniques to help her stay in the present moment. She learns techniques like body scan and mindful breathing (see Chapter 7 for more on mindfulness).
- **Self as context:** The therapist helps Mia understand that she is more than her thoughts. She remembers all the other important things about herself, like her love for dance and her great sense of humour.
- **Values:** Mia and the therapist discuss what is important to her, such as spending time with her friends, doing well at school and feeling happy. They talk about how she can still pursue these values even though her father is in prison.
- **Committed action:** Mia sets small goals for herself to help her live according to her values. For example, she might decide to draw a picture for her father every week.

Critical question

- How could you use DBT or ACT techniques to support your practice?

Theory of Mind (ToM) and mentalising

Theory of Mind (ToM) (Premack & Woodruff,1978) is a fundamental concept in developmental psychology and cognitive science, referring to the ability to attribute mental states (such as beliefs, desires, intentions and emotions) to oneself and others. This capacity enables individuals to understand that others have thoughts and feelings different from their own. ToM is crucial for social interactions, empathy and effective communication, as it allows people to predict and interpret the behaviour of others.

The development of ToM typically begins in early childhood and progresses through several stages. According to seminal research by Premack and Woodruff (1978), children as young as three years old begin to exhibit a basic understanding of the mental state of others. However, it is not until around the age of four or five that children can reliably understand that others can hold false beliefs, an ability often measured by the classic 'Sally-Ann task' (Dennett, 1978). In this task, children are asked to predict where a character (Sally) will look for an object based on her belief (which differs from the child's knowledge of the object's actual location). Successfully predicting Sally's actions indicates an understanding that others can have beliefs that are different from reality as well as different from your own.

Further research by Wellman and Liu (2004) introduced a developmental progression in ToM, suggesting that children first understand diverse desires and beliefs before mastering more complex concepts like false beliefs and hidden emotions. This progression highlights the gradual nature of ToM acquisition and its dependence on cognitive development and social experiences.

ToM is linked to several cognitive and social abilities, including executive function, language development and empathy. Studies have shown that children with better executive function skills, such as working memory and inhibitory control, tend to have more advanced ToM abilities (Carlson et al., 2004). Language development also plays a critical role, as conversations about mental states with caregivers and peers help children internalise and understand different perspectives (Harris et al., 2005).

The importance of ToM extends beyond childhood, influencing social interactions and relationships throughout life. For instance, individuals with high ToM abilities are often better at navigating social complexities, understanding social cues and resolving conflicts. Conversely, impairments in ToM can lead to significant social challenges, as observed in individuals with autism spectrum disorder (ASD). Baron-Cohen et al. (1985) proposed that deficits in ToM could explain many of the social difficulties experienced by individuals with ASD, such as trouble in understanding others' emotions and intentions.

Moreover, ToM is not static and can be influenced by several factors, including cultural contexts and social environments. Cross-cultural studies have shown that while the developmental trajectory of ToM is similar across cultures, the specific age at which children achieve certain milestones can vary (Liu et al., 2008). This suggests that cultural practices and social interactions shape the development of ToM.

As Eirian points out in the case study below, it is imperative that, before commencing any cognitive therapy with a child, the child has an understanding of what thoughts are and how they differ from feelings. Exploring ToM and mentalising (the act of thinking about your own and others' mental states) (Gilead & Ochsner, 2021) can be important first steps in cognitive therapy.

REFLECTIVE TASK

This activity aims to help readers reflect on and enhance their understanding of cognitive approaches to support children's wellbeing through the analysis of a specific case study.

For this activity you will need a notebook, pencil and a quiet, comfortable space for reflection.

Select a case study from your practice experience or create a fictional scenario involving a child who is experiencing emotional or behavioural challenges. Ensure the scenario is detailed enough to provide ample material for reflection.

Write a detailed description of the scenario. Include information about the child's background, the specific challenges they are facing, their demeanour, relationships, behaviour and any interventions that have been tried so far.

Use the following prompts to guide your reflection on how cognitive approaches could support the child in the case study:

- **Understanding the child's perspective:** How might the child's thoughts and beliefs be influencing their emotions and behaviours? What cognitive distortions or negative thought patterns could be at play? What role does ToM play in this process?

- **Cognitive techniques:** Which cognitive techniques (for example, cognitive restructuring, mindfulness, problem solving) could be most beneficial for this child? How would you implement these techniques in your interactions with them?
- **Other strategies:** What other strategies could complement the cognitive approaches to support the child's wellbeing?
- **Measuring progress:** How would you measure the effectiveness of the cognitive interventions? What signs of improvement would you look for in the child's behaviour and emotional state?
- **Emotional support:** How can you give the child emotional support while implementing cognitive approaches? Reflect on the importance of building a trusting relationship and validating the child's feelings.
- **Action planning:** Based on your reflections, write down one or two specific actions you will take to apply cognitive approaches in your practice. This could include trying out a new technique, seeking additional training or setting aside time for regular self-reflection.
- **Ongoing reflection and learning:** These are key to becoming more effective in supporting children's wellbeing through cognitive approaches. Revisit your reflections regularly and continue seeking opportunities for development in this area.

This activity aims to deepen your understanding of cognitive approaches and their impact on children's wellbeing, fostering a more mindful and effective practice.

Practical ideas for using cognitive approaches to support children

- **Thought detective game:**
  The objective is to help children identify and challenge negative thoughts by playing a detective role. Provide each child with a notebook and pen. Explain that they are going to become thought detectives and investigate their own thoughts. Explain that sometimes we all have thoughts that make us feel upset, scared or angry. As a thought detective, their job is to find out if these thoughts are true and helpful.

  Each child thinks about a recent time when they felt anxious or upset, then they write down the thought they had in that moment. The children then investigate the thought, gathering evidence that supports or contradicts its validity. They can write or draw their evidence in their notebooks. Children then challenge the thought, by analysing the evidence they have gathered. Is the thought true, or is there another way of looking at it? The adult can help them produce more balanced or positive thoughts. Finish the game by asking the children how it felt to be thought detectives, what they learned and how they could use these skills in the future. The game can be made more fun with detective hats and magnifying glasses.
- **Coping skills collage:**
  The objective of this activity is to teach the children different coping strategies. Gather materials such as scissors, glue, magazines and a poster board. Ask the child to cut out

the pictures that represent different coping strategies (for example, talking to a friend). Tell them to create a collage. This can be used as a visual reminder of coping strategies for use when feeling overwhelmed.

- **Positive thoughts jar:**
  This can promote positive thinking and self-esteem. Identify a jar for holding positive thoughts. This can be decorated or personalised as required to make it special. Label it 'Positive thought jar'. Provide small paper shapes and pens for the child to record positive thoughts, affirmations or things for which they are grateful. Periodically read the notes together and discuss them.

Case study: a conversation with Eirian (E) and Natasha (N) from MyST

In developing the following case study, I had the privilege of talking to youth worker Natasha Powles and Eirian Teague (an integrative psychotherapist), who both work for MyST (My Support Team), an intensive support service for children, young people and families, based in the South Wales valleys.

Alison: So, tell me about your service.

N: We are a psychology-led, multi-disciplinary service where we offer therapeutic approaches to children and families that are care-experienced, or on the edge of becoming looked after. Our main focus is to rehabilitate children from care, or to prevent family breakdown in the first place.

We develop bespoke packages of care for children and families and offer consultations to support social work locality teams. One of the hallmarks of our service is exceptionally low caseloads, so the work is very intensive.

E: We offer a 24-hour on call service to our families, so we are there when we are most needed.

N: We are not confined to one model of support; rather it is led by the needs of and preferences of the family. It is as if we have a toolbox of many strategies within the therapeutic context, and we can dip into them and use the bits that we think are relevant for each young person.

E: We draw on a whole range of approaches and interventions, but using third wave cognitive approaches is often where we see real breakthroughs for the families. However, we never go straight to those approaches; rather our focus initially is on relationship building, and holding the family safe. It may be months down the line before we can bring in cognitive approaches.

N: There are a lot of considerations when working with children and families. Consistency and reliability are so important. It's all about creating a sort of contract of expectations. We respect boundaries and if something comes up, but the family don't want to go there, we encourage them to tell us, and then we can discuss it. It's not about us enabling avoidance, it is more about giving them the ownership of how and when we address those issues.

E: We recognise that as professionals, there can be all kinds of power imbalances in our relationships with the families, and we believe that it is important for us to reflect on that and find ways to share that power. It is important for us to recognise that for many of the parents we work with, when professionals have come through the door previously, it was often to tell them that they are not good enough, and this was often followed by massive repercussions in the family. So it is important that we humanise the situation of our being there for them. It is also important that we show humility, and when we get something wrong, we own the responsibility, and also model the repair to that relationship.

(Eirian reflected on an on-call conversation when she was woken abruptly from sleep and responded to a parent's question with another question because she was tired and not clear about what was needed. The response did not land well, and immediately, Eirian found herself needing to work towards repairing the rupture, whilst modelling humility and self-reflection.)

N: The team have all been trained in dyadic developmental psychotherapy (DDP), an approach based on principles of attachment and intersubjectivity that is designed to enable traumatised children to trust their caregiver in order to turn to them for comfort and support. Hence it is crucial that the practitioner models healthy patterns of relating and communicating, in order to foster feelings of safety and connection. (Natasha emphasises the importance of case reflection meetings for holding yourself and one another accountable within this context.)

E: Flexibility and adaptiveness are so important. I may have a goal in mind for the session, but it is important that I work responsively and tune into the child, and just drop in my planned input when it is helpful to do so.

N: Yes I agree. I'm thinking of a young person I worked with who was keen to learn the DBT skill of mindfulness. She wanted to be outside, so I took my planned session out into the landscape. We were walking along the lakeside and up a mountain whilst practising DBT skills. It was far more effective than the times we had tried things indoors. It allowed the young person time to reflect and she realised why she was having so many difficulties at school. She learned better in an outdoor context whilst being active.

E: A recurrent theme in my work is helping children to understand what they think and that other people think differently. It is important for children to develop that theory of mind; to understand what a thought is and how it is formulated, and to slowly begin to appreciate that feelings are different from thoughts. There are some great activity worksheets that ask you to do things like colour in feelings, but we find that sometimes the children and young people we work with need a stage before that. And if we miss that earlier stage the intervention is not as effective.

N: It is also important that when a child experiences a difficult feeling like sadness, we just allow them to sit with it, and there is no need to move them on. I think sometimes we steer clear of the difficult feelings because they feel challenging for us and we don't like to think of a child having those feelings, but it is an important part of their processing.

E: Yes and it is where resilience is built. I think that one of those areas of experience versus inexperience is knowing when to allow those moments to just happen. Silence is so powerful and you haven't got to fill it.

E: Cognitive theory work helps people understand that there's a choice. And it's not inevitable. Lots of people think that this has to happen because this did, or will this now happen because I've done this? But we are showing them that even if nothing else changes, you can think differently today. What would it be like to think differently? It's a really hopeful side of the work, even at the times where it's really difficult to hold hope. Whatever else goes wrong, your thoughts are the power that you will retain. How can you think more if you've never seen more? Some people I've worked with struggle to imagine what something better is like, because they haven't experienced it. So being able to construct a place in their mind that gets to be their own and different, something that they own, can help start to offer the chance to think differently.

N: So, it's almost like alongside the therapeutic approach, we almost need to be able to paint a picture of what it would feel like if, for example, you had a job full-time. What would be different in your day? How would it feel? And as practitioners we almost need to lead that kind of visualisation for those we work with who seem stuck in their circumstances.

E: Cognitive restructuring. We had a lovely example of this. A child had been told that she was not able to return home that night. She went to the water tray outside our building and asked for a brush. She just swept the water down into the drain. Just sweeping, sweeping, sweeping, it. And it was almost like a process she had to go through by herself. We didn't intervene, just let her have this moment.

N: We reflected on that later, didn't we, and said how many people would have been tempted to get stuck in and intervene. When she had finished she said her only worry was that she didn't have her special toy and may not be able to sleep without it.

E: She had processed the whole experience and of course we were able to get the toy for her.

N: I suppose a drawback is the can of worms that you can open with child or a family. I've had a child come to me and I was almost certain I knew where the trauma lay. I had the chronology and I had all the information and they tell you a story and it fits. And then the relationship develops. And then along comes the tin opener and then suddenly the trauma that you thought it was has shifted to another area and you think, "Oh my goodness, I didn't plan for this."

E: It is important that we know what we don't know, and that we don't wade in where angels fear to tread. I think, Do I have the expertise for this?, or Do we need more specialist help here? That is important because inadvertantly an untrained person stepping into a specialist area can do harm.

N: Yes, and also, our own self-care is crucuial. It's not just having a bath or going for a walk. It is self-compassion. So I think it's pitching it carefully, and not not keeping yourself safe to a degree that it inhibits the work. But knowing off limits as well.

Because if you face burnout, it will have implications for yourself and others.

E: Yes, professional humility, self-care, self-compassion and self-reflection – that's what helps us in what we do.

Critical questions

- Eirian and Natasha stress the importance of professional humility in our work with families. What does this term mean to you and how do your practise it?
- In the example of the child at the water tray, how was the self-motivated water play helping her to process difficult thoughts and feelings. What lessons are there for practice in this example?
- Eirian talks about "knowing what you don't know", knowing the limits of your experience and training and being prepared to seek specialist support when it is needed. Why is this so important? In your role, how do you make use of specialist services to support children and families?
- "Self-care, self-compassion and self-reflection" – what do you understand by these terms and how do you practise them?

Conclusion

This chapter has explored the important contribution that talking therapies can make to supporting children and families. It is important to recognise that talking therapies are not an approach that works for everyone, and the practitioner needs to be cognisant of the age, development and preferences of the child when considering the most appropriate support they can provide. Of all the approaches explored in the book, it is this one that requires most additional training in order to safely and ethically use the techniques. With the knowledge and understanding provided in this chapter, non-specialist practitioners can signpost to specialist services to support children's wellbeing. It is, as Eirian points out in the case study, important that "we know what we don't know", and "do not wade in where angels fear to tread". However, there is also potential to use some of the ideas provided to help children in their immediate situations. As with all other approaches, building a trustful and empathic relationship is fundamental to this.

Talking therapies: key points

- Prior to any intervention, it is essential to build a trustful therapeutic relationship with the child or young person.
- Common factors, such as the skills, knowledge and empathy of the practitioner, are as important in ensuring a positive outcome as the intervention itself.
- These approaches work best when children and young people display high levels of engagement and commitment to the process. This is particularly important in the case of home-based practice.
- Talking therapies, particularly CBT-based approaches, are really helpful **tools** for supporting children and young people's wellbeing. However, they are not a suitable approach for very young children, some children with developmental challenges or children in a crisis situation.
- Whilst these approaches demand a trained and registered practitioner for their effective delivery, many of the techniques can be adapted for more general use.

ADDITIONAL RESOURCES

- The NHS website (www.nhs.uk/mental-health)

This is a great first point for accessing reliable information about mental health conditions and wellbeing in general. All materials are based on the most up-to-date evidence available. There are helpful signposts to further support and information.

- Young Minds Website (https://www.youngminds.org.uk)

This website has a helpful range of resources about children's mental health and wellbeing, specially designed for young people and parents, as well as extensive materials to support practitioners.

- Stallard, P. (2019) *Think good, feel good: a cognitive behavioural therapy workbook for children and young people*. London: John Wiley & Sons.

This is a very practical and helpful workbook containing a range of ideas and helpful resources for practitioners.

References

Baron-Cohen, S., Leslie, A.M. and Frith, U. (1985) Does the autistic child have a "theory of mind"? *Cognition*, 21(1), pp. 37-46.

Carlson, S.M., Moses, L.J. and Claxton, L.J. (2004) Individual differences in executive functioning and theory of mind: an investigation of inhibitory control and planning ability, *Journal of Experimental Child Psychology*, 87(4), pp. 299-319.

Clark, D.A. (2013) Collaborative empiricism: a cognitive response to exposure reluctance and low distress tolerance. *Cognitive and Behavioral Practice*, 20(4), pp. 445-454.

Clark, D.A. (2020) *The negative thoughts workbook: CBT skills to overcome the repetitive worry, shame, and rumination that drive anxiety and depression*. Oakland, CA: New Harbinger Publications.

Creswell, C., Waite, P. and Hudson, J. (2020) Practitioner review: anxiety disorders in children and young people – assessment and treatment, *Journal of Child Psychology and Psychiatry*, 61(6), pp. 628-643.

Dennett, D.C. (1978). Beliefs about beliefs, *The Behavioural and Brain Sciences*, 1(4), pp. 568-570.

Dippel, A., Brosschot, J.F. and Verkuil, B. (2024) Effects of worry postponement on daily worry: a meta-analysis, *International Journal of Cognitive Therapy*, 17(1), pp. 160-178.

Dolan, N., Simmonds-Buckley, M., Kellett, S., Siddell, E. and Delgadillo, J. (2021) Effectiveness of stress control large group psychoeducation for anxiety and depression: systematic review and meta-analysis, *British Journal of Clinical Psychology*, 60(3), pp. 375-399.

Gilead, M. and Ochsner, K.N. (2021) A guide to the neural bases of mentalizing, in *The neural basis of mentalizing*. Cham, Switzerland: Springer International Publishing, pp. 3-16.

Greimel, K.V. and Kröner-Herwig, B. (2011) Cognitive behavioural treatment (CBT), in Møller, A.R., Langguth, B., De Ridder, D. and Kleinjung, T. (eds.) *Textbook of tinnitus*. New York: Springer, pp. 557-561.

Harris, P.L., de Rosnay, M. and Pons, F. (2005) Language and children's understanding of mental states, *Current Directions in Psychological Science*, 14(2), pp. 69-73.

James, A.C., Reardon, T., Soler, A., James, G. and Creswell, C. (2020) Cognitive behavioural therapy for anxiety disorders in children and adolescents, *Cochrane Database of Systematic Reviews*, 11(11). doi: 10.1002/14651858.CD013162.pub2.

Kidd, S.A., Davidson, L. and McKenzie, K. (2017) Common factors in community mental health intervention: a scoping review. *Community Mental Health Journal*, 53, pp. 627-637.

Leahy, R.L. (2008) The therapeutic relationship in cognitive-behavioural therapy, *Behavioural and Cognitive Psychotherapy*, 36(6), pp. 769-777.

Linehan, M. (2014) *DBT? Skills training manual*. New York: Guilford Publications.

Liu, D., Wellman, H.M., Tardif, T. and Sabbagh, M.A. (2008) Theory of mind development in Chinese children: a meta-analysis of false-belief understanding across cultures and languages. *Developmental Psychology*, 44(2), pp. 523-531.

NHS (2024) Types of talking therapies. Available at: https://www.nhs.uk/mental-health/talking-therapies-medicine-treatments/talking-therapies-and-counselling/types-of-talking-therapies (Accessed 1 October 2024).

NHS (n.d.) 5 steps to mental wellbeing. Available at: https://www.nhs.uk/mental-health/self-help/guides-tools-and-activities/five-steps-to-mental-wellbeing (Accessed 1 October 2024).

Premack, D. and Woodruff, G. (1978) Does the chimpanzee have a theory of mind? *Behavioural and Brain Sciences*, 1(4), pp. 515-526.

Prowle, A. and Hodgkins, A. (2020) *Making a difference with children and families: re-imagining the role of the practitioner*. London: Bloomsbury Publishing.

Sakdalan, J.A., Shaw, J. and Collier, V. (2010) Staying in the here-and-now: a pilot study on the use of dialectical behaviour therapy group skills training for forensic clients with intellectual disability, *Journal of Intellectual Disability Research*, 54(6), pp. 568-572.

Wellman, H.M. and Liu, D. (2004) Scaling of theory-of-mind tasks, *Child Development*, 75(2), pp. 523-541.

9
The power of stories

Introduction

Stories have always been an important feature of human culture, used to pass on learning and understanding. However, stories offer more than a channel for communication and can embody profound therapeutic value. Through narratives, individuals can process emotions, make sense of experience, find meaning in the complexities of life and connect with others. This chapter explores several ways in which stories and storytelling can be used by practitioners to support children's wellbeing. We also consider the potential of stories to support practitioners' reflection and professional development.

The therapeutic value of stories

As Perrow (2012) points out, all stories have the power to be therapeutic. She argues that the process of listening to a story (regardless of its content) can be healing. However, Perrow also notes that specific stories employed in specific contexts can have a therapeutic value that goes beyond the generic potential of stories to calm and heal. Such stories can be employed very purposefully by the practitioner to bring about therapeutic outcomes. Engaging with carefully chosen or constructed narratives can enable children to express feelings that are difficult to articulate, gain new perspectives and foster resilience. Hence, storytelling can promote healing and self-discovery, providing comfort, understanding and hope in times of distress (Sunderland, 2017). Below are some of the therapeutic benefits of storytelling for children.

- **Comfort in times of change:**
  Even as adults, many of us have a favourite book or film that we go to when times get tough. For me (Alison), Little *House on the Prairie* (book or TV series – I am not fussy!) is something I reach for when I need to escape current hardships. The vivid storytelling immediately exports me to a place where I can lose myself in the narrative and feel warm and safe. Familiar stories can offer comfort during times of stress or change; the predictability and structure of a well-known, much-loved story provides a sense of stability, and helps children to feel secure and reassured.

- **Naming, understanding, and processing difficult feelings:**
  Stories can provide children with a way of identifying and expressing the emotions characters are experiencing. With the help of a story children can better understand their own feelings and experiences which helps them process difficult emotions like fear, sadness and anger. Through narratives that depict characters overcoming challenges children can learn about perseverance, problem solving and the idea that difficulties can be overcome. This helps build resilience and gives them tools to face their own challenges
- **Fostering empathy:**
  Stories often depict a variety of perspectives and situations allowing children to metaphorically step into the shoes of others. This increases their ability to empathise with people from different backgrounds or situations and understand the impact of their actions, which is essential for developing healthy social relationships.

Bibliotherapy

The word bibliotherapy comes from two Greek words: *biblio* (book) and *therapeia* (healing). Bibliotherapy, therefore, is a therapeutic approach that involves the use of books and reading materials to help children understand and manage various emotional and psychological challenges. It is a versatile tool that can be adapted to suit different age groups, developmental stages and individual needs. At its core, bibliotherapy employs the power of stories to provide children with a safe space to explore their feelings, experiences and social situations. The narrative within the book serve as a mirror reflecting the child's own experiences, and as a window offering perspectives on situations that they may not have encountered personally (Pardeck & Pardeck, 2021). This dual function helps children to develop empathy, self-awareness and problem-solving skills.

The process of bibliotherapy typically begins with the selection of appropriate literature that resonates with the child's particular circumstances. This could range from dealing with common childhood issues like fear of the dark, or making new friends, to more complex topics such as dealing with loss, divorce or trauma (Jensen, 2020). The selected book serves as a starting point for discussions between the child and the parent/practitioner. Through guided discussions, children are encouraged to express their thoughts and feelings about the story and relate it to their own experiences. They can also explore workable solutions to their problems. One of the key benefits of bibliotherapy is its non-threatening nature (Ginns-Gruenberg & Bridgman, 2021). Unlike direct forms of therapy, where children may feel uncomfortable or resistant to discussing their issues, bibliotherapy allows them to approach these topics indirectly through characters and situations in a story. This can be particularly beneficial for children who are shy, introverted or reluctant to open up about their feelings as the story provides a buffer zone, giving the child the emotional distance needed to engage with difficult topics without becoming overwhelmed (Sunden, 2023).

Moreover, bibliotherapy can enhance cognitive development by improving literacy skills, expanding vocabulary and fostering a love for reading. When children engage with stories, they not only learn to navigate their emotions but also develop critical thinking and comprehension skills, analysing characters and motivations. Understanding the plot and predicting outcomes helps to build cognitive abilities that are essential for academic success (Sara *et al.*, 2024).

Additionally, bibliotherapy can be tailored to address specific cognitive or learning challenges such as ADHD or dyslexia by the selection of books that are accessible and relevant to the child's experience (Alvarez, 2023).

Another significant aspect of bibliotherapy is its role in promoting social and cultural awareness. Through diverse stories, children are exposed to different cultures, lifestyles and viewpoints that can broaden their understanding of the world and foster inclusiveness. This exposure helps to develop empathy and social skills as children learn to appreciate differences and make connections with others (Heath et al., 2023).

Bibliotherapy is a very versatile approach that can be implemented in various settings including homes, schools and clinical environments. It can be used as a standalone intervention or to complement other therapeutic approaches. Bibliotherapy is a powerful tool that can help to foster resilience and support social development. By providing children with the opportunity to see themselves in stories and explore solutions in safe and engaging way, bibliotherapy help them feel empowered to navigate the complexities of their world with confidence and empathy. It is, therefore, a valuable and versatile tool for the practitioner's therapeutic toolbox.

Using stories therapeutically

Over the last 20 years or so, a plethora of stories have been published with the specific purpose of helping children explore and understand challenging situations and difficult emotions. These books often have a very sound therapeutic foundation, a character the child can identify with, a compelling storyline and a message of hope. Practitioners can build their own small library of books, get to know the book well and provide toys and activities to make the story come alive (De Vries et al., 2017). It is important for practitioners to choose books that are culturally relevant and age appropriate; in general terms, it needs to be a good fit with the developmental stage of the child. Moreover, knowing the child well will enable the practitioner to tune into the child's current interests and enthusiasms.

However, there is a degree of trial and error in this as we never quite know which stories will resonate with a child. The example below, drawn from my own practice experience, highlights this point.

 Practice vignette

In 2017, I (Alison) was working at the children's centre in a refugee camp in northern France. I had taken with me several story sacks based around well-known stories, with resources included in the bags to help bring the story alive, especially for children for whom English was an additional language. One morning, I was reading *The Gingerbread Man* to a small group of children aged 4-6, when I noticed a much older child hovering at the edge of our story circle and listening attentively. When the activity ended and the other children went off to make gingerbread cookies, I had the chance to work on a one-to-one basis with this child, a 12-year-old boy from Kurdish Iraq, who had arrived in the camp a few weeks previously, after a hazardous journey with his mother and siblings. He was keen for me to read the story to him again and again, whilst he joined in with the refrain "Run, run as fast you can. You can't catch me, I'm the Gingerbread Man". Over the course of the next week, the story provided opportunities for dramatic retellings, artwork and den building. At the end of the week, the Children's Centre manager noted that the boy's emotions seemed much more regulated, and that he was building positive relationships with the Centre staff and other children. When I left the camp, the boy kept the knitted gingerbread toy as his very own pocket pal.

Critical question

- How did the gingerbread man story provide a vehicle for exploring the child's difficult experiences of migration?

In this case, the story that really resonated with the boy was one aimed at a much younger audience. However, the Gingerbread Man running from danger and surviving despite the odds (in this version at least!) chimed with his own experience and provided a safe space for exploring and validating emotions, talking about difficult experiences and building connections with others. Using puppets, animals and artefacts connected to the story all help build engagement. Activities where the child can make and keep something connected to the story can extend the learning and provide a visual reminder with longevity (Noonan-Lepaon & Ridgway, 2009). It goes without saying that stories should be culturally appropriate, and it is helpful for the child to see aspects that are related to their own experience; this might include characters of a similar age or, ethnicity or facing similar experiences and family situations. However, as the example above showed, we cannot always predict the connections and meanings that the child will derive from the book. Books with characters that are non-human (for example, animals) can also be extremely successful in engaging children and young people.

The practice vignette above looked at how stories can highlight aspects of children's own lived experience, helping them to make sense of what they have encountered and to feel less alone with the big emotions they are feeling. However, as well as reflecting aspects of our own experience, stories can also be used to help children enter into the experiences of others. This can help foster empathy and understanding of other children's lives and support the inclusion of marginalised others.

 Case study: Sue Barrow, *The Power of Stories*

In the case study below, young adult author, Sue Barrow, explores this important aspect of bibliotherapy.

Why stories?

> Stories have always been used to pass on learning and knowledge. A good story, written or told aloud, has the power to pique our curiosity and engage our imagination and

understanding. Stories can stop us in our tracks, keep us reading well into the night and stay in our heads long after the final page. We have all read them! In this case study we will consider the impact reading stories has on children and young people. Stories that transport them into lives they have never lived, be it a boarder at Malory Towers, a child stepping through a wardrobe and finding themself in Narnia or a thoughtful spider helping her piglet friend escape the chop!

The subjects I write about in my novels for teens and young adults are those that deal with contemporary social issues. Known as realistic fiction, this is a genre which focuses on relatable characters coping with real-life issues. Real life can be so many things – funny, sad, exciting, scary, wonderful, awful and sometimes extraordinary and terrifying. If it is presented in an honest, sensitive and responsible way, there is little that is off-limits in young adult fiction. Of course we must take our characters on a roller-coaster ride, testing them to within an inch of their lives. And when their chances of happiness seem slim, we pull something out of the hat to offer hope and a way forward. This is how the best stories are crafted.

My first novel, Keeping Secrets, features Ceri, a gangly, 16-year-old redhead who finds herself feeling out of place and increasingly unhappy in her adoptive family. Lacking a sense of identity, she secretly pursues a journey of discovery about her early life only to find that it leaves her with more questions than answers. Searching a few years later for another 'issue' to get my teeth into, I hit on – quite by accident – a newspaper report covering the trial of a UK professional couple accused of trafficking a young girl into their home and using her as a domestic slave. Child trafficking was a crime that I had never heard of. Parents in poverty are tricked into sending their children abroad on the false promise of a better life. It sounded horrific. Straight away I knew this was a subject I had to write about. A story that would keep readers on the edge of their seats but at the same time help them understand and become better informed about this particular issue of social justice.

The power of storytelling had never seemed more critical. It seemed unlikely that my novel would make even the tiniest dent in this appalling trade in lives. But written as a thriller – exciting, engaging and well researched – might make young people sit up and take notice, even get involved in the fight against trafficking. And so Sold was born, with my main character, Roza, a bright, 15-year-old living in poverty in Albania, suddenly offered the prospect of a better life in the UK. When she arrives, she discovers this is a lie. Her father has sold her into slavery to get out of debt. Forced to work as an unpaid servant, beaten and abused, Roza does not think life can get much worse… until she escapes.

Stories, therefore, can help children understand societal issues by weaving themes of family strife, adoption, bereavement and loss into the plot, unlike in fantasy or science-fiction genres. Bringing child trafficking into my storylines has given me the opportunity to raise awareness of this issue, to educate, evoke empathy and spark discussion.

Helping develop empathy and understanding

Books play a significant role in building empathy in children and young people. Those who read regularly are more inclined to be empathetic, tolerant of different viewpoints and able to engage with others on an emotional level. This in turn fosters their own wellbeing and resilience. Research has shown that children are more likely to absorb the message through a fictional story than reading facts and figures; more likely to remember the details too, and for longer. Most novels have a main character. Studies show that children relate more readily to an individual – to their personal story, their character traits, their strengths, and weaknesses – than to an amorphous group. This in turn builds emotional intelligence, creating a bond between the reader and the main character, allowing the reader to root for the main character and empathise with whatever troubles they are going through. For example, in Keeping Secrets – Ceri's concern for the plight of homeless people in the Welsh Valleys over time translates to compassion for her birth mother whom she fears may have suffered the same fate after a spell in prison. In Sold, the reader may well think Roza has enough problems of her own to deal with when she ends up at the Cannabis Farm. However, although she is irritated by the behaviour of her fellow-slave, Hanna, she understands how badly her asthma affects her, shows her kindness and helps her escape.

Reinforcing moral values

Stories also have a role in teaching or reinforcing moral values: the difference between good and evil, the importance of kindness, loyalty and understanding. In Keeping Secrets, for example, Fran stays loyal to her best friend, Ceri, even though she does not agree with her searching for her birth mother. In Sold, the harsh realities of trafficking are highlighted by the 'good guys' who reach out to Roza in her struggle for freedom.

Developing Imagination

Another benefit of story-reading is the development of the reader's imagination. Transported to different worlds, children may find themselves questioning some of the actions or decisions the main character takes in pursuit of their goal. They may find themselves examining the way the character gets themself out of sticky situations (or not!) and suggest different problem-solving skills. They might even imagine a different ending from the one written! In Keeping Secrets, for instance, Ceri and her best friend Fran fall out. In Sold, Roza's stubborn, determined-to-do-things-her-own-way streak leads her to reject offers of help.

Creating rapport and recognition of a shared humanity.

Realistic fiction *allows us to investigate another's life. It enhances our understanding about them and creates common ground. The best stories may evoke a sense of kinship and shared humanity, bridging the gap between our diverse backgrounds and finding common threads that bind us together. This is shown in Keeping Secrets, when Ceri struggles with her identity, has questions about her past and a longing to understand who she is. In Sold, Roza is an ordinary young woman with her own hopes and dreams, who becomes caught up in the extraordinary and appalling world of human trafficking.

Denied the most basic human rights (safety, freedom, food, clothing and education), she also battles the ignorance of trafficking, the shame of it (in her eyes) and not being believed. Her gutsy approach to her circumstances, driven by her determination to win her freedom, can be an inspiration to readers.

Helping children understand and make sense of their own experiences

Readers find comfort and resonance in stories that mirror their own struggles. For a child struggling with their identity, either through adoption or being in care, reading about Ceri's (Keeping Secrets) sense of having landed in the 'wrong' family because of her height and shoe size might resonate strongly (if not for those reasons).

In Sold, Roza's experiences may resonate with those who have fled war-torn countries, immigrants and asylum seekers. For children, reading works much like role-playing, allows them to see the world through someone else's eyes. When readers identify with a character, they understand that others are also experiencing and coping with personal struggles just as they are. Keeping Secrets and Sold both feature characters who, in turn, feel sad, lonely and scared and are not afraid to admit it. They give way to their feelings through confusion, frustration, tears, anger and low moods. In very differing circumstances Ceri and Roza both have to adjust their expectations of the future and recognise the need to find a way to forge new paths ahead.

In summary, the power of stories is immense. It is central to understanding ourselves and our place in the world, and how we engage with others.

Therapeutic benefits for me as a writer

I was no stranger to creative writing when I decided to bring Ceri and Roza to life in my two realistic fiction stories. A childhood scribbler, I could often be found penning outlandish tales or writing detailed accounts of my first trip to London aged 12! I love writing, bringing characters to life in stories and situations I care about. Writing about real life, particularly young people, and the struggles they endure either due to the circumstances they have been born into, or the actions of adults over which they have no control, is important to me. My words will resonate with someone going through a similar experience. Others may be helped to better understand a world outside theirs and empathise.

It feels like a worthwhile use of my time. It makes me feel fulfilled. Particularly when it came to writing Sold. Trafficking was beyond my power to control, I knew that. But writing a book about it was not! Sitting in front of my laptop and typing words on to the page freed me up to have a real sense of agency.

Critical questions

- Sue suggests that stories are more powerful than bald facts in helping children to grapple with difficult issues. Do you agree? Can you think of examples from your own reading that have stayed with you and/or shaped your thinking about a particular issue?

- Sue highlights several therapeutic and educational benefits of using books with children. How can you harness these benefits within your own practice?
- Sue explains the therapeutic benefits she experiences from writing. To what extent might creating their own stories provide similar benefits for children?
- Sue talks about how writing fosters a sense of personal agency. How can stories (both those written by others and those developed by children themselves) support children's own sense of autonomy and agency?

Developing our own stories

Whilst "off the shelf" books can be extremely useful, children benefit particularly from creating their own narratives (Moula, 2021). This gives the child real ownership over the story as well as unleashing their creativity and individuality. The child has autonomy to decide where the story starts, how it moves forward and how the characters are portrayed. Stories can be created in written form, in pictures or using digital multimedia. Santos *et al.* (2020) even explore the use of chatbots in enabling children to develop narratives that explore feelings. Again, the practitioner can adapt their approach to the individual child and employ all sorts of approaches to support the child's creativity. Over the years my own practice has used story dices, story prompts, play dough, puppets and found objects to beneficial effect. In today's technologically advanced world, there is enormous scope for children to create their own multimedia or digital stories.

REFLECTIVE TASK

Think about a child that you have worked alongside who has experienced some form of loss. Research age-appropriate books that you could use to support the child. Spend time familiarising yourself with one book. Consider how you would use the story with the child:

- How would you identify a conducive environment for sharing the story? How would you introduce it?
- How might you engage the child with the story?
- What activities might you pair with the reading to enrich the child's experience?
- How could you support the child to relate the themes to their own experience?
- What strategies would you use to help the child process their emotions?
- How would you follow up this activity?

You may wish to journal about you experience of this reflective activity.

Life story work

A particular form of story making with children is the life story approach. The purpose of life story work is to share ideas, feelings and information that help the child create a real understanding of their own life journey, experiences and identity (Hammond *et al.*, 2020). Often, life stories are created for or with children who are being adopted but can have positive benefits for other children with complex life histories. A wide range of people can contribute to the creation of a child's life story, for example, children and young people, foster carers, birth family members, social workers and teachers. Hence, when completed sensitively and effectively, a life story can help create a rich picture.

However, Baynes (2008) stresses the importance of practitioner reflection and ethicality within life story work, emphasising the importance of creating a narrative that is respectful of the family. She also explores notions of practitioner power and the importance of developing trustful, authentic and democratic relationships with children when engaging in life story work.

Some different approaches to life story work

Life story work can follow a narrative pattern, drawing upon key events and milestones in the retelling. However, another approach is to use a more symbolic approach. The approaches below have been used successfully with our undergraduate students, helping them to experience and understand the value of life stories for reflection and personal development.

Me in a box

This reflective activity provides students or children with the opportunity to gather or create artefacts that represent their life and place them in a shoebox. The box can then be decorated appropriately. In small groups, students use their boxes to tell the story of their life. The choosing of the artefacts allows them to emphasise the aspects of their story that are meaningful to them, and that they are willing to share. This is a non-threatening activity that allows the child much autonomy, is fun to make and meaningful to keep.

Kawa River Model

The Kawa River Model (Iwama, 2011) is a therapeutic method developed in Japan by occupational therapists based around the metaphor of life as a river (*kawa* in Japanese). The imagery follows a river's course, from its source in the mountains until it flows into the ocean. As it follows its meandering path, the river's flow will vary according to events and environment. There will be boulders (challenges) that limit its flow for a time, but also driftwood (assets) that support the river's flow. Students can draw or make representations of their river and conversations with the practitioner can help them think about how to overcome challenges and maximise assets.

The Tree of Life

Like the Kawa River Model, the Tree of Life (Ncube, 2006) is an inspiring approach to working with children and young people who have experienced adversity, this time using the metaphor of a tree. Originally the Tree of Life approach was developed from Zimbabwean folklore to support children affected by HIV/AIDS in southern Africa. However, the universal imagery of a tree with roots, branches, leaves and fruit has resonance way beyond its original context. Children begin by drawing a tree and then consider its constituent parts. The tree imagery can then be used to tell stories about their life, explore difficulties and find solutions.

The beauty of these three approaches lies in their flexibility, as they can be adapted for children of all ages, abilities and backgrounds. The activities work equally well on a small group basis or when working one-to-one.

> **Critical questions**
>
> - What qualities does the practitioner need in order to effectively use bibliotherapy?
> - What ethical considerations should be taken into account when using bibliotherapy?
> - Are there any potential challenges or limitations related to using bibliotherapy in our work to support children and families?
> - How might you enhance your use of stories within your own therapeutic work?

Storytelling as a tool for reflection and personal development

Storytelling can be a powerful tool for reflection and professional development as it helps practitioners make sense of their experiences and learn from them in a meaningful way. There are several ways in which storytelling can assist the reflection process.

- It can help us organise our experiences through retelling the situation, whether it was a challenge, a mistake or something that went well. This approach is especially useful in thinking about critical incidents. It can help a practitioner to think about what happened, why it happened and what the outcome was. This process of organising and verbalising our thoughts helps clarify our experiences, making them easier to analyse.
- Retelling the story can help us gain perspective, allowing us to take a step back and view our experiences from different angles. By thinking about how others might perceive the same event, or by framing the story in diverse ways, we can gain new insights and a broader perspective on our actions, decisions and their consequences.
- The storytelling process can help us learn from experience. Reflecting on our own stories helps identify what worked well and what did not, so we can learn from both success and failure. Such reflection is key to professional growth as it allows us to consciously apply these lessons in future situations.
- Reflective stories can be useful in building emotional intelligence. Sharing stories often involves discussing emotions, both our own and those of others involved. This practice can serve to make us more aware of our feelings and the impact they have on our work. It also fosters empathy as we explore the experiences of others.
- Storytelling provides opportunities for peer learning. When we share our stories with colleagues, it opens up opportunities for collective reflection and learning. Others can offer their perspectives, share similar experiences and provide feedback, which can lead to deeper insights and more effective professional development.

Over time the stories we tell about our career can help us to see our own development. By reflecting on past stories, we can track how our skills, thinking and professional identity have all evolved, which reinforces the sense of progress and motivation. From critical incident reflections to identifying and sharing moments of professional joy and triumph, storytelling offers unique opportunities for individual and collective growth and development.

Conclusion

In the course of this chapter we have considered the importance of books and stories as a means of exploring difficult issues, understanding our own and others' experiences and building empathy and resilience. We have explored the value of using stories that already exist and of creating our own stories. As practitioners, we have also considered the importance of careful planning when choosing and using books, to provide the most benefit for children we work with. Finally, we have contemplated reflective writing as a means of making sense of our professional experiences and contributing to our own development. Books are an invaluable resource for the therapeutic practitioner toolkit.

The power of stories: key points

- Bibliotherapy refers to the use of books as a therapeutic tool to help support wellbeing.
- Stories can be used to foster empathy, to help understand our own emotions and to provide inspiration and hope.
- Creating their own stories can help children to express themselves, communicate emotions and experiences and connect with others.
- Writing is a useful tool for the practitioner to support their own critical reflection.

ADDITIONAL RESOURCES

- Rees, J. *Life story work with adopted children*. Available at: https://firststeps.first4adoption.org.uk/exercises/life-story-work

This video explores the benefits of life story work from the perspective of an experienced practitioner.

- Barrow, S. (2006) *Keeping Secrets*. Llandysul: Pont Books.
- Barrow, S. (2023) *Sold*. Bournemouth: Cadence Publishing.

These are the books discussed in the case study.

- The Book Trust. Available at: https://www.booktrust.org.uk/booklists/t/picture-books-to-help-you-talk-about-tough-topics.

The Book Trust is a reliable source for practitioners. It has helpful articles as well as suggestions for suitable books to use with children facing adversity. The page above contains some excellent picture books that can be used therapeutically.

- Empathy Lab UK https://www.empathylab.uk

The Empathy Lab is a social enterprise developed to help foster empathy among children. It includes resources to support practitioners as well as recommended books for supporting children's empathy.

- Gillie Bolton, *How about Writing?* Available at: https://www.gilliebolton.com/?page_id=161

This is a useful website for practitioners wanting to explore the benefits of reflective writing. The website contains helpful videos and resources as well as examples of Gillie's own writing.

References

Alvarez, A.D. (2023) Teaching mindfulness skills using bibliotherapy to address ADHD symptoms in children, Doctoral dissertation, Azusa Pacific University, Los Angeles.

Baynes, P. (2008) Untold stories: a discussion of life story work. *Adoption & Fostering*, 32(2), pp. 43-49.

Bolton, G. (1999) *The therapeutic potential of creative writing: writing myself*. London: Jessica Kingsley Publishers.

Bolton, G. (2006) Narrative writing: reflective enquiry into professional practice. *Educational Action Research*, 14(2), pp. 203-218.

Brown, E. (2012) *Loss, change and grief: an educational perspective*. London: David Fulton Publishers.

De Vries, D., Brennan, Z., Lankin, M., Morse, R., Rix, B. and Beck, T. (2017) Healing with books: a literature review of bibliotherapy used with children and youth who have experienced trauma. *Therapeutic Recreation Journal*, 51(1), pp. 48-74.

Ginns-Gruenberg, D.D. and Bridgman, C. (2021) Using bibliotherapy as a catalyst for change, in Kaduson, H.G. and Schaefer, C.E. (eds.) *Play therapy with children: modalities for change*. Washington, DC: American Psychological Association, pp. 75-92. https://doi.org/10.1037/0000217-00.

Hammond, S.P., Young, J. and Duddy, C. (2020) Life story work for children and young people with care experience: a scoping review. *Developmental Child Welfare*, 2(4), pp. 293-315.

Heath, M. A., Cutrer-Párraga, E.A. and Young, E.L. (2023) Classroom bibliotherapy to support social emotional learning: increasing inclusion, kindness, and understanding of diversity, in Alberton Gunn, A. and Bennett, S.V. (eds.) *Teaching multicultural children's literature in a diverse society*. New York: Routledge, pp. 20-37.

Iwama, K.H.L.M.K., 2011. The Kawa (River) Model, in Duncan. E.A.S. (ed.) *Foundations for practice in occupational therapy-E-BOOK*. London: Elsevier Health Sciences, p.117.

Jensen, L. (2020) The effects of bibliotherapy on students experiencing grief, loss, and trauma. *Counselor Education Capstones*, 133. Winona State University. Available at: https://openriver.winona.edu/counseloreducationcapstones/133.

Moon, J. (2001) Learning Teaching Support Network (LTSN) Generic Centre PDP working paper 4: reflection in higher education learning. *Higher Education Academy*, pp. 1-25.

Moula, Z. (2021) "I didn't know I have the capacity to be creative": children's experiences of how creativity promoted their sense of wellbeing. A pilot randomised controlled study in school arts therapies. *Public Health*, 197, pp. 19-25.

Ncube, N. (2006) The Tree of Life project. *International Journal of Narrative Therapy & Community Work*, 1, pp. 3-16.

Noonan-Lepaon, F. and Ridgway, A. (2009) Story sacks: look what is inside! *An Leanbh Óg, The OMEP Ireland Journal of Early Childhood Studies*, 3(1), pp. 89-98. Pardeck, J.T. and Pardeck, J.A. (2021) *Bibliotherapy: a clinical approach for helping children*. Abingdon: Routledge.

Perrow, S. (2012) *Therapeutic storytelling*. Stroud: Hawthorn Press.

Santos, G.A., De Andrade, G.G., Silva, G.R.S., Duarte, F.C.M., Da Costa, J.P.J. and de Sousa, R.T. (2022) A conversation-driven approach for chatbot management. *IEEE Access*, 10, pp. 8474-8486.

Sara, A., Keyvan, S., Soheila, K., Hasan, S. and Noruzi, A. (2024) Building self-esteem in elementary school students: the promising benefits of bibliotherapy. *Informology*, 3(1), pp. 127-142.

Sunden, S. (2023) Storytelling and bibliotherapy: tools and techniques for children receiving therapeutic intervention. *Journal of Poetry Therapy*, 37(1), pp. 1-12.

Sunderland, M. (2017) *Using story telling as a therapeutic tool with children*. Abingdon: Routledge.

Part III
Enhancing the role of the practitioner in supporting children and families

10
The attuned practitioner

Introduction

Attunement is the ability to be aware of, and responsive to, another person's emotions and needs. It is a way of recognising and responding to an individual's moods, words and actions, and is intricately linked to emotional attachment. To be emotionally attuned, someone must be fully present and actively listen to others. This chapter considers the importance of attunement for practitioners working with children and families. Barriers to attunement are examined with consideration of how we can become more attuned. The chapter critically explores a range of theoretical concepts and models, including approaches to listening, unconditional positive regard and attachment theory.

The attuned practitioner

Writing in a clinical context, Erskine (1998) describes attunement as a

> kinesthetic and emotional sensing of others, knowing their rhythm, affect and experience by metaphorically being in their skin, and going beyond empathy to create a two-person experience of unbroken feeling and connectedness by providing a reciprocal effect and/or resonating response.
>
> (p.236)

Dr Dan Siegel (2007) suggests that children need attunement in order to develop well and to feel secure. This need for attunement continues throughout our lives, helping individuals to feel connected to others and understood.

Attunement is more than simply showing awareness or empathy. Rather, it is about connecting with another person's emotional state, understanding their needs and responding appropriately, in a way that they feel understood and valued. The word 'attunement' always reminds me of the process of tuning in to a radio station on a non-digital device; it requires patience and a sensitive touch as we seek to align the frequencies to get the best reception. Attunement, therefore, requires conscious effort and practice. It entails being fully present, in the moment, paying close attention to non-verbal cues and responding with empathy and understanding. This may mean putting aside our own distractions and preconceptions in order to truly listen and observe. It requires patience and a willingness to step into another person's emotional world without judgement or the urge to fix things immediately. Hence attunement is not just something that we do but is an essential part of who we are as practitioners. A key aspect of attunement is the ability to regulate one's own emotional responses. In high stress or conflict situations it can be challenging to remain calm and empathic. However, maintaining an attuned disposition requires self-regulation and emotional intelligence. It is important to be aware of one's own emotional triggers and to manage them in a way that allows for a compassionate and constructive response to others (see Chapter 11 for more on this). When working with children who have experienced difficulty, an attuned practitioner can help create a safe and supportive environment that facilitates emotional safety and development.

Attunement is important from birth. An attuned carer will go beyond addressing the basic needs of a child such as feeding or changing but will begin to tune into the baby's emotional needs. Hence, they will recognise when a cry signifies hunger, discomfort or the need for emotional comfort and will respond appropriately, providing not just physical care but emotional support. As children grow older, attunement continues to play a crucial role in their development. By paying attention to a child's verbal and non-verbal cues, listening actively to their words and observing body language, an attuned practitioner will validate the child's feelings and open communication channels, allowing the child to express their emotions without fear of judgement. It is important to recognise that attunement is not just about responding to difficult emotions, it is also about celebrating positive ones. Hence, the attuned carer or practitioner will share a child's excitement about a new accomplishment or a fun experience, mirroring the child's enthusiasm, showing genuine interest and enjoyment. Such positive reinforcement helps build the child's self-esteem and encourages them to continue their exploration and self-expression.

Biemans (1990) identified several principles of attunement. These principles consider how emotions are expressed and received within human interactions. Kennedy *et al.* (2011) built on this, with research involving the close study of interactions between mothers and young infants. The following principles were identified:

- **Being attentive:** This might involve turning towards the person, looking towards them and making eye contact, looking interested, using nods, encouraging intonations, adopting a friendly and non-threatening pose, using proximity or giving them space as needed. For the practitioner, being attentive will also involve choosing a time and place where you will not be interrupted and making a conscious decision to leave aside other concerns in order to attune.
- **Actively listening:** This may involve being emotionally available and positive, waiting for a response and being comfortable with short silences. The practitioner needs to remember that much of communication is non-verbal. Mehrabian (1971) famously asserted that 7 per cent of communication takes place through the words we use in spoken communications, while 38 per cent takes place through tone and voice and the remaining 55 per cent of communication takes place through the body language we use and most specifically, our facial expressions. Hence the attuned practitioner needs to be cognisant of all these factors.

- **Receiving:** This involves beginning to repeat or reflect back what you heard to show that you have listened, matching and mirroring body language to encourage them to open up further, using their words rather than professionalised versions of their words, and 'wondering aloud' to further explore thoughts and feelings. For the practitioner, the wondering aloud can be a helpful, non-threatening and non-directive way of enabling the child to move towards more positive possibilities.
- **Being attuned together:** This entails bringing the conversation onto a more equal and cooperative footing, by taking turns to talk, sharing thinking and feelings, regularly checking for understanding. This stage can be particularly helpful in enabling the child connect their thinking and feelings with their behaviour if they have not already done so.
- **Guiding and supporting:** This step may involve simplifying things to make them more understandable, exploring ideas, alternatives or choices, problem solving or providing more information or practical help. It is important to remember that if we bypass the initial stages and jump straight to giving guidance and support (which practitioners may be tempted to do when juggling multiple priorities) then we have not truly attuned to the child.
- **Deepening discussion:** At this stage, if we are attuned to the other person and we have a trusting relationship, we can use activating questions to stimulate the other person's thinking and address their thoughts and assumptions. We can also voice our own opinions and demonstrate that people can disagree respectfully, which may be particularly helpful in situations where conflict has not been managed well.

These principles are helpful in helping us to reflect on our own attunement, and in doing so, focus on ways in which we can better support children and families.

Attunement and attachment theory

One of the key benefits of attunement is the development of secure attachment (see Chapter 3 for more on attachment theory). Children who experience attuned caregiving learn to trust that their needs will be met, and that their emotions are important. This sense of security lays the foundation for healthy emotional regulation and positive and interpersonal relationships. However, where previous attachments have been less secure, resulting in anxious, avoidant or disorganised attachment patterns (Ainsworth 1978) the attuned practitioner can model a supportive and inclusive response by tuning into the child, recognising that they are struggling or feeling disengaged, and respond with interest, care and compassion. Hence, it is helpful for the practitioner to assess early relationships, where the information is available, and observe the child's behaviour and emotional responses to identify patterns that may stem from attachment issues. It is then important to create a secure and safe environment through conscious and consistent attunement. Over time, creating a trusting relationship with the child through active listening and empathy will help to validate the child's feelings and experiences. Through such attunement, the child can then learn to understand and express emotions, find coping strategies and have healthy and positive relationships modelled to them.

REFLECTIVE TASK

Find a quiet and comfortable place at a time when you will not be disturbed. It would be helpful to have journalling materials to hand. This activity is designed to help you think more deeply about attunement and to explore how attunement feels to someone on the receiving end of it.

Defining the experience

- Think about a time when you felt truly understood, seen and heard.
- Describe the experience in as much detail as you can recall. What was the situation and who was involved?

Emotional processing

- How did it feel to be seen and heard in that moment?
- Describe the emotions you experienced.
- How did this feel in your body?

Understanding the experience

- Can you remember any specific words or actions that contributed to making you feel understood and seen in that moment?
- Was it body language, tone of voice or something that was said?
- Why do you think this experience stood out for you?
- What made it different from other interactions?

Connection and trust

- How did the experience affect your relationship with the person involved?
- Did it strengthen the bond between you or build trust?

Self-knowledge

- What did you learn about yourself from this experience?
- Did it change the way you perceive yourself or your needs?
- How can you create more moments where you and those around you feel understood, seen and heard?

Practice

- What can you do to foster these kinds of connections within your practice?

The professional artistry of listening

Listening is more than simply auditory processing. It involves empathy, presence and understanding. At its core, this skill involves fully engaging with the speaker; not just hearing their words, but also tuning into their emotions and underlying messages. Effective listeners create a safe space where individuals feel valued and understood, fostering trust and open communication. It is a form of professional artistry. This artistry requires the listener to be mindful, setting aside their own judgements and distractions to focus entirely on the speaker. By reflecting back what they hear, and asking thoughtful questions, listeners can uncover deeper insights and facilitate more meaningful dialogue. This practice enhances interpersonal relationships and helps to build trust.

Behaviour as communication

Rogers (1995, p.91) famously said, "We speak with more than our mouths. We listen with more than our ears." An important aspect of attunement involves viewing children's behaviour as a form of communication (see Chapter 3 for more on behaviour as communication). Immediately, asking ourselves what a child's actions and demeanour may be saying about their emotional state moves us away from just responding on a surface level to the behaviour we are observing. An angry outburst may signify a child's frustration or a need for attention. Similarly, a child withdrawing may indicate fear or anxiety. Even positive behaviours such as sharing a toy may point towards the child's need for connection or social approval.

Attunement as engagement of Head, Heart and Hands

Pestalozzi (2022) first introduced the notion of Head, Heart and Hands as an holistic approach to children's learning. However this principle can be equally applied to practitioners' work with children. To really tune in to a child, therefore, we need our professional listening to encompass our head, hear, and hands (Gazibara, 2013). This will result in authentic and holistic attunement (see Chapter 3 for more on Head, Heart and Hands). In this context the **Head** represents the knowledge and understanding that practitioners bring to their interactions with children. It is crucial that practitioners understand child development and are knowledgeable about the many ways in which children communicate their needs. Practitioners will then use their knowledge to observe and interpret children's behaviours accurately. The **Heart** symbolises the emotional connection and empathy required for attunement. Practitioners show compassion towards the child and remain emotionally present throughout the interaction. This will involve active listening, validating the child's feelings and responding with warmth. Through these means, children will feel understood, valued and secure. The **Hands** refer to the practical application of attunement in daily interactions. This includes the actions and strategies that practitioners use to support children's needs effectively, for example, comforting a distressed child, setting up routines that provide stability or planning activities that promote positive relationships.

Critical questions

- How can practitioners effectively observe and interpret non-verbal cues to ensure that they are attuned to the emotional and psychological needs of children?
- How can attunement practices be adapted to support children with diverse backgrounds and varying attachment styles?
- How does the concept of attunement extend beyond the child to influence their interactions with family dynamics, peer relationships and educational settings?
- What are the potential challenges practitioners might face when trying to establish attunement with children and how can these be overcome?
- Can you think of a time when you have intentionally employed attuned responsiveness with a child? What was the outcome?

The practice vignette below illustrates a practitioner intentionally attuning to a child who is experiencing frustration.

 Practice vignette

Amira is a seven-year-old girl who recently went into foster care. She has been displaying challenging behaviours at school since her arrival there three weeks ago. Amira often disrupts lessons, has frequent outbursts and struggles to follow instructions. The teaching assistant working with her class, Rob, has noticed that Amira's behaviour seems to escalate during transitions and group activities. One afternoon, during the group art project Amira becomes frustrated when she cannot find the colour she needs. She starts shouting and throws the pencils on the floor. The children look startled, and the classroom becomes tense. Rob, who has been learning about attuned responsiveness as part of his foundation degree programme, approaches Amira calmly. He kneels to Amira's level and speaks softly, "Amira I can see that you're feeling really upset right now. It's OK to be frustrated. Can you tell me what's bothering you?" Amira, still upset, looks at Rob and starts to cry, "I can't find the blue pencil. I need it for my sky!" Rob says, "I understand. It sounds like the blue pencil is important for your picture. Let's take a deep breath together and see if we can find it." After a few deep breaths, Amira and Rob look for the pencil, which they find under another table. Rob says, ""Here it is. I'm glad we found it. How about we work on your sky together for a bit?" Amira is feeling calmer now, and she nods. Rob stays with her for a few minutes, offering encouragement and support. Amira begins to focus on her work and her frustration subsides. Later, Rob reflects on the situation. He realises that by acknowledging Amira's feelings and providing a calm presence, he was able to help Amira regulate her emotions. He decides to incorporate more check-ins with Amira during transitions and group work to prevent future outbursts. Over the next few weeks Amira's behaviour improves. She still has moments of frustration but with Rob's attuned support she learns to express her feelings more constructively. The classroom environment becomes more positive, and Amira begins to enjoy participating in group activities.

Critical questions

- In what specific ways did Rob demonstrate attuned responsiveness towards Amira?
- How does Rob apply a head, heart and hands approach to supporting Amira?

Unconditional positive regard (UPR)

'Unconditional positive regard' (UPR) is a term coined by Carl Rogers, a humanistic psychologist. The concept, much used within human services, refers to accepting and valuing a person without any conditions. Fundamentally, UPR is about creating an environment where an individual's worth is not measured by achievements or behaviours, but solely by their existence. When applied to children, UPR has profound positive implications for their emotional and psychological development. For children (and indeed adults) such acceptance can be transformative.

Young children are constantly learning about themselves and the world, taking cues from those around them. When children consistently experience UPR from their caregivers, they develop a stable sense of self-worth (Brown et al., 2009). This unconditional acceptance acts as a stable foundation on which they build a positive sense of identity (Guteman, 2020). Hence, one of the most important benefits of UPR is the enhancement of a child's self-esteem. When children feel unconditionally valued, they are more likely to take risks, explore their interests and engage in creativity (Daniel, 2020). In this context, children are not afraid of failure because they know that their worth is not tied to success or perfection. This can lead to a more resilient and adaptive personality, capable of navigating the challenges of life with confidence (Proctor, 2022).

In practice, adopting a UPR stance would entail embodying a belief that all children are intrinsically special, unique and worthy of professional love and respect. It means recognising that for a variety of reasons, a child may well display behaviours that are not considered acceptable, but the child is always accepted, valued and included. Hence, even when a child makes mistakes or exhibits challenging behaviour, they are not made to feel unworthy or unloved. Instead, the focus is on understanding the underlying reasons for their actions and guiding them towards positive behaviour (Gordon, 2017). To put this important learning into context, let us explore another practice scenario.

 Practice vignette

Eleven-year-old Emma has been observed bullying some younger girls at an after-school club. Saima is the club's manager. Saima previously worked in a context where behaviour was managed using a system of rewards and sanctions. In this context, Emma's behaviour would have led to an immediate sanction, such as missing out on a fun activity or having time out. Her parents would also have been contacted.

However, Saima is keen to apply UPR on this occasion. She sits down with Emma and begins to talk about the situation. Saima stresses that she wants to understand what is going on and find ways to help. Initially Emma is very defensive, and avoids eye contact, but Saima maintains a warm and non-judgemental demeanour. Saima acknowledges that it must be hard for Emma to deal with so many emotions and asks what it is that she feels might be making her act that way. After some hesitation Emma begins to talk about feeling isolated and misunderstood, which has made her lash out at others. Saima acknowledges Emma's feelings and thanks her for sharing her feelings with her. Emma feels heard and respected. Saima has succeeded in separating Emma's behaviour from her worth as a person. Now Saima explains that Emma's behaviour is not the best way to handle those feelings. Together they work on finding other ways to express feelings and build better relationships with the rest of the group. Nothing is better immediately, but Saima's approach has enabled Emma to feel valued and supported, whilst also helping her to think about more appropriate ways of coping with her uncomfortable emotions. Over time a consistent UPR approach helps Emma to become part of the group and begin to enjoy her time at after-school club.

Critical question

- How does Saima demonstrate UPR towards Emma, and what difference does this make?

UPR helps foster a powerful sense of security and trust in relationships. When children know they are accepted no matter what, they are more likely to open up about their feelings, fears and experiences. This open communication is crucial for their emotional development and helps build stronger adult-child bonds. It also teaches children to extend the same level of acceptance and empathy to others, promoting healthy social interactions (Testa, 2022).

We would argue that UPR is a foundational principle for effective work with children and families. It has universal application across professional disciplines and practice contexts. Whilst it should be applied to all children and young people we encounter in practice; it is perhaps most powerful when used with children who have had previous experience of not being loved and accepted unconditionally. In such contexts, it can be transformative and can ultimately enhance children's sense of their own worth. In essence, UPR is about offering children a safe psychological space where they are free to grow, explore and become their authentic selves. It is a profound way of valuing and supporting children, ensuring they develop into emotionally healthy and confident individuals. Through UPR, we affirm the inherent worth of every child, laying the foundations for more compassionate and enabling practice.

 Case study: Antoinette Frearson (Part 2)

In Chapter 2 readers were introduced to Layla, a child facing considerable adversity. Here, we consider how Antoinette responded to Layla's needs.

> When I started working at the special school Layla had already been there for a term. In my first lesson with her, I observed that she was quiet, tense and on high alert. Her eyes

moved all around the room, taking in any little noise and she seemed to jump whenever someone spoke, or the door opened. I also noticed that she held some toys in her clasped hand. This state of hyper-alertness left her completely disengaged from the lesson and unresponsive to any instructions or direct requests. Consequently, she struggled to complete any tasks given and when the teacher began to reprimand her, she would panic and flee the room. Support staff would need to follow her, for her safety, but it felt like a game of cat and mouse. He rans around the school grounds, I could hardly keep up with her. Finally, she would stop running, the adrenaline and fear all spent, and when I arrived close behind, she would curl herself up into a foetal position, crying and unresponsive to me, despite any efforts to discuss how she was feeling, what made her flee the room or requests to return to the lesson. During break times, Layla seemed like a different person. She would run around the playground in circles. Being outside was an evident release to her, and she seemed genuinely happy. It was a fragile happiness though, because if a fellow student was unkind to her, she would run away and look for certain staff for connection. She would sit outside the staffroom or their classroom doors in the foetal position and wait for them.

Layla was regularly receiving lunchtime detentions for non-compliance. She would bring toys into school she would not relinquish when asked to, and she was extremely sensitive to any peer comments or negativity of any kind. So, it seemed clear to me that Layla was still struggling with her past and this was having a massive impact on her present. She found learning a near impossibility, she was struggling to socialise and make meaningful connections with her peers and she was continually getting on the wrong side of the teachers as she was not engaging or complying and therefore not making any progress.

Up until this point, the school had been "managing Layla's behaviour" with a behaviour plan and a sanction system. The sanctions were applied progressively if the behaviour did not change. As a result, Layla was having a negative experience of school. From my postgraduate study, I had done a lot of reading around disorganised attachment disorder, challenging behaviour, mentoring and coaching, as well as the effects and impacts of early life adversity and neglect in children. The literature I had read not only gave me a different viewpoint but also some confidence to subtly challenge practice. I was keen to explore an alternative approach, which was recognising Layla's trauma and her emotional needs. Not wanting to criticise colleagues, I engaged them in discussions about Layla's wellbeing, but it was clear that staff had differing views. Table 10.1 summarises some of these discussions.

At breaktime, a colleague would say, "Layla is sitting by the staffroom door crying for you. Just ignore her." I could not because thus far that is what she had experienced all her life. To ignore her would reinforce this view of the world that no-one is there for here and no-one answers her cries for help. So, I would get up and I would sit with her and listen to her. That was the substitute experience she was looking for. If she were not eating at lunchtime, I would reassure her the food was hers to eat if she were hungry. I would then 'check-in' with her from time to time, so she knew she was being seen and heard but there was no drama. I would take a note of what she ate (or did not) and would message her mum just to let her know. I left her food in front of her until she left the table, as taking food away could trigger a deep memory.

Table 10.1 Perspectives on taking a therapeutic approach to a child experiencing a disorganised attachment

Staff perspectives	An alternative interpretation
'She can be clingy, so you must be strict with her. Do not give into her neediness!'	She had been diagnosed with disorganised attachment disorder because of the neglect she had experienced in her early life. Some of these symptoms include the child wanting the caregiver then moving away when the caregiver responds, fearful facial expressions, appearing as if they're in a trance and being disoriented (Paetzold et al., 2015). In view of this she may need a substitute experience; someone who she can form a healthy attachment with and trust. Someone who is consistently there for her (Skynner & Cleese, 1983) rather than someone who supports her then withdraws from her – this could be perpetuating what she has already experienced.
'She may refuse food at lunchtimes. Take away the food if she is not eating it. Do not rise to the behaviour, it is just another attempt at attention-seeking.'	She was starved and neglected previously. Reassure her that the food is hers to eat if she is hungry. Do not remove the food from her as this may be a trigger of previous experience (NSPCC, 2021).
'Her younger sister is fine, goes to mainstream school, is well-adjusted and is achieving age-related expectations. She just cannot be bothered to work.'	She has struggled more than her sister because she was older, more aware and had endured her experiences for longer (Brodzinsky et al., 2022).

> She seemed to live in survival mode and a constant state of hyper-alertness. To reduce her anxiety and increase feelings of safety and relaxation, I implemented some relaxation and calming strategies whenever possible and attempted to engage her using her special interests (Social Care Wales, 2022.
>
> I bought an anxiety self-help book for children. It was entitled What to do when you worry too much by Dr Dawn Huebner. It included short cognitive behavioural therapy (CBT) techniques, analogies and age-appropriate discussions on anxiety. In a fortnightly enrichment lesson, which she struggled to cope with, we would sit in the library and work through the book. She would then take the book home to show her mum the exercises we had worked through, and her mum told me it gave her valuable insight into Layla's worries and concerns.
>
> During lessons and following the use of a calming or relaxation strategy, I would engage her by using her special interests of horse-riding and swimming to access the work. I also developed a new intervention plan which included staff being cognisant of Layla's emotional needs and seeing her 'behaviour' as a form of communication. I used literature to share my trauma awareness with the staff team, particularly providing opportunities for recovery by forging new positive neural pathways and integrating more helpful coping strategies. I explained that children's brains are different from adult brains which are harder to rewire and reconfigure due to more established brain circuitry (Center on the Developing Child, 2007). I am delighted to say that the plan was approved by a supportive senior leadership team and cascaded to all school staff.

Over the course of that year there were small incremental improvements in Layla's behaviour. Within the new supportive atmosphere, she was able to become more resilient with peers and more self-aware of her feelings. Her independence slowly grew. Her struggles around food remained but seemed to reduce as emotional recovery increased. She became more skilled at handling her own anxiety by implementing learned strategies and mindfulness techniques. This enabled her to engage in lessons and she rarely fled from the classroom. She left school with some qualifications and is now enjoying college. Her rehabilitation will be lifelong and as previously stated, it will not be a linear journey, but recovery is happening.

Reflecting on my journey I have realised the following:

- *Developing a more therapeutic approach for a student takes time, patience and requires resilience.*
- *You need to be realistic in your expectations; recovery may not happen despite your and the school's best efforts, but this does not mean that the approach is not worth implementing.*
- *Throughout the journey, record what you are seeing so you can measure the positive impact and identify patterns in negative behaviour which will inform the most effective techniques and areas that still need addressing, such as environmental barriers.*
- *Lastly, but most importantly, keep self-care at the top of your daily to-do list. 'Putting your oxygen mask on first' is not selfish, it is essential. You can only fill your student's emotional cup if your tank is full.*

Change may not be easy and there are no quick fixes to long-term mental health recovery but making a positive difference to a child's life that will have lifelong effects on their wellbeing and potential will always be worth the effort, energy and input. Good luck!

Critical questions

- Antoinette paints a vivid picture of how Layla was struggling at school. The behaviour plan and sanctions system worked well for many other children. Why was this approach less successful with Layla?
- Antoinette recognised that behaviour is a form of communication. What are some of the things Layla is communicating? How could an attuned practitioner respond?
- Antoinette, as a new member of staff, was very keen to avoid alienating or criticising colleagues, whilst still advocating for the rights of the child in this demanding situation. What strategies did she adopt in order to make a real change for the child?
- Antoinette grounds her approach in theory. From your reading, what have you learned about being an attuned practitioner?

Setting the scene for attunement

It is important that practitioners give thought to creating an environment that is conducive to wellbeing and developing a trustful relationship. Ideally, this environment will be welcoming, non-threatening and free from distractions. The outdoors can provide a wonderful setting for building relationships and facilitating meaningful interaction (World Health Organization, 2017) (see Chapter 6 for more on the benefits of the outdoors). Meeting in open, outdoor spaces can permit an authentic, human-to-human encounter, whilst also experiencing the known benefits of being in the natural world (British Psychological Society, 2020). However, indoor spaces can also provide an opportunity for wellbeing and connection. Some settings will have access to a nurture room, the aim of which is to improve the emotional wellbeing of children and young people who may be struggling. The nurture room provides a comfortable environment where children feel safe and relaxed. It is designed to be a homely, warm and welcoming space where the emphasis is on emotional safety; it enables a safe base for children with reliable adults, clear boundaries, empathic language and non-punitive approaches (Boxall, 2013). In some settings it may be more manageable to create a 'cosy corner,' an oasis of calm and cosiness that children can retreat to, based on the Danish concept of *hygge* (Prowle & Hodgkins, 2016). Blankets, cushions, fleeces and faux fur throws can be used to make a warm snug area where children can relax. There should be no electronic devices present, just books and pictures to look at in peace. Texture and feel are especially important, with many Danish settings having a dog or cat for children to stroke. Soft lighting and furnishings contribute to the peaceful and nurturing quality of the space.

Dyck (2002) suggests that creating a nurturing environment involves paying attention to six elements: aesthetic, space, light, noise, colour and temperature. A warm and welcoming aesthetic encourages communication and connection. Jarman (2013), who developed the notion of communication friendly spaces, notes that open spaces are considered emotionally unsafe for a child, whereas smaller and more private spaces can encourage the feeling of safety and give the child confidence. Keeping noise levels low promotes focus and calmness.

However, as important as the physical environment is the creation of conditions for connection. The physical environment does not compensate for the relationship with trusted adults and the quality of interactions between those adults and children and young people.

Conclusion

This chapter has explored the importance of attuned responsiveness within our work to support children and families. Attunement is both a disposition we can embody and a skill to practise and continually hone. It is through such attunement that we will develop trustful and authentic relationships with the children and families we work with and create an emotional environment that is conducive to providing effective support. However, it is important to acknowledge that working with others in this way is emotional labour (Winter *et al.*, 2019), which can take its toll on practitioners' own wellbeing. Hence, it is imperative that practitioners prioritise their own self-care, which is the focus of the next chapter.

The attuned practitioner: key points

- Attunement is how we 'tune in' to another's thoughts, feelings, and responses. It requires being emotionally present, focused on the other person and ready, willing, and able to listen.
- The quality of our attunement is something we can practise and improve. This will have benefits for our practice but also for other interpersonal relationships.
- Adopting a position of UPR is a useful starting point for attunement.
- All behaviour is communication. The attuned practitioner will look beyond the surface to what the behaviour may be saying about the individual's thoughts, needs or feelings.
- Attunement is emotionally demanding. Self-regulation is an important aspect of attunement. Practitioner's attention to their own wellbeing and self-care is vital.

ADDITIONAL RESOURCES

- Beacon House website https://beaconhouse.org.uk.

This website, which was developed by clinical psychologists, has an extensive range of resources and information related to trauma, attachment and attunement.

- *Attunement in the Age of Technology: TED talk by Dr Gwennyth Palafox*. Available at: https://www.youtube.com/watch?v=OIbL7b9sf7Q.

This is a thought-provoking, 20-minute talk about attunement against a backdrop of increasing technology in all aspects of our lives.

- Faber, A. and Mazlish, E. (2012) *How to talk so kids will listen and listen so kids will talk*. London: Simon & Schuster.

This popular book, written for parents by educationalist and parenting experts provides a highly readable and thought-provoking introduction to aspects of attunement.

References

Ainsworth, M.D.S. (1978) The Bowlby Ainsworth attachment theory. *Behavioural and Brain Sciences*, 1(3), pp. 436–438.

Biemans, H. (1990) Video home training: theory method and organisation of SPIN, in Kool, J. (ed.) *International seminar for innovative institutions*. Ryswijk, Netherlands: Ministry of Welfare Health and Culture, pp. 96–112.

Boxall, M. (2013) The nurture group in the primary school, in Bennathon, M. and Boxall, M. *Effect intervention in primary school*. Abingdon: Routledge, pp. 18–38.

British Psychological Society (2020) *The use of talking therapy outdoors*. Available at: https://cms.bps.org.uk/sites/default/files/2022-09/Use%20of%20talking%20therapy%20outdoors.pdf (Accessed 30 October 2024).

Brodzinsky, D., Gunnar, M. and Palacios, J. (2022) Adoption and trauma: risks, recovery, and the lived experience of adoption. *Child Abuse & Neglect*, 130, Part 2, doi: https://doi.org/10.1016/j.chiabu.2021.105309.

Brown, G.L., Mangelsdorf, S.C., Neff, C., Schoppe-Sullivan, S.J. and Frosch, C.A. (2009) Young children's self-concepts: associations with child temperament, mothers' and fathers' parenting, and triadic family interaction. *Merrill-Palmer Quarterly*, 55(2), pp. 184–216. doi: https://doi.org/10.1353/mpq.0.0019.

Center on the Developing Child (2007) *The science of early childhood development (in brief)*. Available at: https://developing.child.harvard.edu/inbrief:thescienceofearlychildhooddevelopment (Accessed 2 January 2024).

Daniel, G.R. (2020) Safe spaces for enabling the creative process in classrooms. *Australian Journal of Teacher Education*, 45(8), pp. 41–57.

Dyck, J.A. (2002) The built environment's effect on learning: applying current research. *Montessori Life*, 14(1), pp. 53–56.

Erskine, R.G. (1998) Attunement and involvement: therapeutic responses to relational needs. *International Journal of Psychotherapy*, 3(3), p. 235–244.

Gazibara, S. (2013) "Head, heart and hands learning" – a challenge for contemporary education. *The Journal of Education, Culture, and Society*, 4(1), pp. 71–82.

Gordon, C. (2017) *Parenting strategies to help adopted and fostered children with their behaviour: trauma-informed guidance and action charts*. London: Jessica Kingsley Publishers.

Guterman, L. (2020) *The progression of parenting and childhood leading to developing an understanding of unconditional self-acceptance*. New York: Hofstra University.

Jarman, E. (2013) *The communication friendly spaces approach: re-thinking learning environments for children and families*. Rye: Elizabeth Jarman Ltd.

Kennedy, H., Landor, M. and Todd, L. (2010) Video interaction guidance as a method to promote secure attachment. *Educational and Child Psychology*, 27(3), pp. 59–72.

Mehrabian, A. (1971) *Silent messages*. Belmont, CA: Wadsworth Publishing Co.

National Society Protection against Cruelty to Children (NSPCC) (2021) Protecting children from neglect. Available at: https://learning.nspcc.org.uk/child-abuse-and-neglect/neglect (Accessed 3 December 2023).

Paetzold, R., Rholes, W. and Kohn, J. (2015) Disorganized attachment in adulthood: theory, measurement, and implications for romantic relationships, *Review of General Psychology*, 27(3). doi: 10.1037/gpr0000042 (Accessed 31 December 2023).

Pestalozzi, J.H. (2022) *The education of man: aphorisms*. New York: Open Road Media.

Proctor, C., (2022) Enhancing wellbeing in youth: positive psychology interventions for education in Britain, *Handbook of positive psychology in schools*. Abingdon: Routledge, pp. 451–465.

Prowle, A. and Hodgkins, A. (2016) Cosy up! *Nursery World*, 25, pp. 15–16.

Rogers, C.R., 1951. Perceptual reorganization in client-centered therapy, in Blake, R.R. and Ramsey, G.V. (eds.) *Perception: an approach to personality*. New York: Ronald Press Company, pp. 307–327. doi: https://doi.org/10.1037/11505-011.

Rogers, F. (1995) *"You Are Special: Words of Wisdom for All Ages from a Beloved Neighbour"*, New York: Penguin Books.

Siegel, D.J. (2007) *Siegel/mindful brain: reflection and attunement in the cultivation of well being*. New York: W.W. Norton & Company.

Skynner, R. and Cleese, J. (1983) *Families and how to survive them*. Oxford: Oxford University Press.

Social Care Wales (2022) *Children who experience trauma*. Available at: https://socialcare.wales/resources-guidance/improving-care-and-support/children-who-are-looked-after/children-who-experience-trauma (Accessed 3 December 2023).

Testa, D. (2022). Supporting vulnerable students: staff and parents speak. *Health Education Journal*, 81(3), pp. 280–292.

Winter, K., Morrison, F., Cree, V., Ruch, G., Hadfield, M. and Hallett, S. (2019) Emotional labour in social workers' encounters with children and their families. *The British Journal of Social Work*, 49(1), pp. 217–233.

World Health Organization (2017) *Urban green space interventions and health: a review of impacts and effectiveness*. Available from www.euro.who.int/__data/assets/pdf_file/0010/337690/FULL-REPORT-for-LLP.pdf?ua=1&utm_source=The%20King%27s%20Fund%20 newsletters&utm_medium =email&utm_campaign=8285918_NEWSL_HMP%202017-05-16&dm_i=21A8,4XLGE, OWYH5H, IQEL 0,1 (Accessed 29 January 2025).

11
Supporting our own wellbeing

Introduction

There is probably a reason why you want to work with children and families who have experienced adversity, something in your personality that makes you super able to connect with others. This is the 'gift' of empathy (Moxley, 2022, p.7) and makes people feel that they can trust you with their worries. It is a privileged position and can be very rewarding. If you do not guard against giving too much of yourself however, it can also be depleting. This has implications for both practitioners and their employers resulting in low job satisfaction, stress, absenteeism and the cost of employing temporary staff (Kusma et al., 2012), which may affect children's development and compromise relationships with families (Bloechliger & Bauer, 2016). This has resulted in more attention being given to the wellbeing of those working with children and families (Bullough & Hall-Kenyon, 2018). In this chapter we discuss how to protect your core self and maintain your wellbeing.

What do we know about wellbeing?

'Wellbeing' is a buzzword vaguely applied to how we feel; 'mental health' and 'wellbeing' are used interchangeably. We cannot be certain whether any measures to improve wellbeing are effective, however, if we do not understand what it entails (Gillett-Swan & Sargeant, 2015).

Dodge et al. compare wellbeing to a seesaw, defining it as "the balance point between an individual's resource pool and the challenges faced" (2012, p.230) further explaining, "stable wellbeing is when individuals have the psychological, social and physical resources they need to meet a particular psychological, social and/or physical challenge. When individuals have more challenges than resources, the see-saw dips, along with their wellbeing, and vice-versa" (Dodge et al., 2012, p.230). So, wellbeing is not fixed but alters dependent on how able we are to cope with our current and past circumstances. Other researchers accept that although wellbeing is fluid, it stays within a constant range and everyone has a "set point" of wellbeing dependent on their genetics (nature), environment (nurture) and experiences (culture), and is therefore person specific (Cummins et al., 2014, p.270). If our wellbeing set point is high, we tend to return to that regardless of our material possessions, finances or location (Royer & Moreau, 2015).

Incorporating wellbeing into the overarching umbrella of health, the World Health Organization (WHO) defined health as "a state of complete physical, mental and social wellbeing and not merely the absence of disease or infirmity" (n.d., para. 14). This demonstrates the interconnected nature of physical wellbeing, mental and emotional wellbeing, social wellbeing and spiritual wellbeing. This definition is useful because it reminds us that being well is holistic and affected by more than a one-off, self-care activity such as taking a bath or going for a walk (Moxley, 2022, p.31).

Mental health

The term 'mental health' has a more clinical meaning than 'wellbeing' and relates to symptoms of mental disorders such as stress and anxiety (Ettema & Schekkerman, 2016). If an individual does not have the resources to cope with their difficulties a specific mental health condition may develop. The WHO (2022) recognised the connection between wellbeing and good mental health, defining mental health as "a state of wellbeing in which the individual realises their own abilities, can cope with the normal stresses of life, can work productively and fruitfully, and make a contribution to their community" (WHO, 2022). This encompasses physical health and wellbeing, for example, chronic physical pain can contribute to low emotional wellbeing and further mental health issues, such as clinical depression.

Wellbeing and the workplace

Sound wellbeing is crucial for good mental health; however, it is not as simple as applying a one-size-fits-all strategy, not least because life is full of ups and downs beyond our control. Sometimes the discourse around wellbeing implies that it is the individual's responsibility to improve their mental wellbeing, which is problematic because much of what affects wellbeing is shaped by social and political systems (Corr *et al.*, 2015). Work-related wellbeing, including employee engagement and job satisfaction, plays a significant role in our overall life satisfaction (Organisation for Economic Co-operation and Development, 2022). Employee wellbeing affects productivity, and workplace culture affects workers' wellbeing (OECD, 2022).

What causes low wellbeing at work?

Working in regulated services always adds pressure to the job; managing parents' expectations and complaints, dealing with inspections, applying for grants and funding, paperwork, covering staff illness and health and safety issues all have the potential to make us feel down. There are, however, other less obvious causes for low wellbeing.

The cost of emotional attunement

Emotional attunement, a deep emotional attachment, enables us to appreciate children's needs and respond appropriately. Young children can sense when a carers' body language does not align with their words, causing them to feel incongruence and uncertainty (Bradford,

2012). Being genuinely attuned, therefore, makes us effective practitioners; however, consider some of the findings of a recent survey of early years practitioners:

- More than two thirds (69%) had cared for babies and young children that were affected by trauma (including child abuse, neglect, the witnessing of violence or involvement in an accident or natural disaster).
- Almost half (49%) said they had cared for children who have experienced the death of a parent or sibling, and 43% reported having looked after children whose family were involved with the criminal justice system.
- 73% reported that they regularly encountered parents who are struggling to manage the emotional, social or mental health needs of their children.
- 91% said they had faced challenging situations at work with young children who they felt were experiencing mental health problems or social or emotional difficulties.
- 86% said they had cared for young children whose behaviour they found particularly challenging, for instance children who were unusually disruptive, disobedient, or hard to control.
- Of the 91% who said they had faced challenging situations at work with young children, over 70% said they felt stressed or upset by these situations and didn't know how best to respond.

(Nelinger et al., 2021, p.4)

These statistics show that working with children and families can be emotionally draining, potentially resulting in

> vicarious trauma, where we soak up young person's past or present trauma. This can become so overwhelming that we begin to experience ... the physical and emotional consequences of it ourselves. We can begin to feel how the young person feels.
>
> Parker, 2020, p.6)

The blurred line between personal and professional

Caring about and for children and families can become such a core part of our identity that sacrificing our own needs for others becomes second nature. Moxley (2022, p.7) writes of "giving away [her] power carelessly" by assuming a responsibility to fix everything, even when unconnected to her role. She considers that this may have been rooted in a desire to prove that she was good enough for the job and an invaluable team member. Eventually, this led to a personal breakdown, and she later reflected,

> Working with children is a big part of who we are ... but it should not be all of who we are.... We often blur the line between personal and professional boundaries without even realising it, working with children is an emotive role that requires us to give so much of ourselves to children and their families and our colleagues.
>
> (Moxley, 2022, p.8)

Compassion fatigue

If we feel emotionally and physically exhausted to the point where we no longer feel empathy for others, we may be experiencing compassion fatigue (Simmons & Wright, 2023), an occupational hazard for those in caring professions because of the frequent exposure to heartbreaking stories. Some have linked it to secondary traumatic stress, whereby you experience trauma after being exposed to the trauma of others (Moxley, 2022). Compassion fatigue is not inevitable, however, and awareness of its signs and symptoms can help prevent this adversely affecting wellbeing.

Burnout

Herbert Freudenberger (1975) developed the term "burn out" after noticing behaviour patterns in himself and colleagues working in community-facing, caring professions. Physical symptoms included:

> a feeling of exhaustion and fatigue; being unable to shake a cold, feeling physically run down; suffering from frequent headaches and gastro-intestinal disturbances; this may be accompanied by a loss of weight, sleeplessness, depression, and shortness of breath. In short, one becomes psychosomatically involved in one or more ailments.
>
> (Freudenberger, 1975, p.74)

The Institute for Quality and Efficiency in Health Care (2000) detailed other symptoms burnt out individuals may experience:

- Alienation from (work-related) activities: the job is increasingly stressful and frustrating. They may become cynical about their working conditions and colleagues. At the same time, they may distance themselves emotionally and feel numb about their work.
- Reduced performance: burnout mainly affects everyday tasks at work, at home or when caring for family members. People with burnout are very negative about their tasks, find it hard to concentrate, are listless and lack creativity.

(Institute for Quality and Efficiency in Health Care, 2020)

Freudenberger theorised that committed and dedicated people find themselves "subtly get(ting) (them)selves into a personal burn-out trap" due to a "three-way squeeze" of demands; intrinsic pressure to succeed, pressure from the people we are trying to help, and pressure from management to produce positive data (Freudenberger, 1975, p.74).

There is a further, related concern for those involved in this "emotional labour" (Hochschild, 1983), the expectation that we will draw on emotions as part of our professional role, for example, continually smiling, which may be at odds with what we feel inside. Commings and Wong suggest that "Limitations on the expression of 'real' feelings or expectations that individuals must display authentic positive emotions can lead to individuals feeling alienated from their own feelings through their commodification as part of their work role", in other words, we become so used to faking emotions as part of our role that we lose touch with what we really feel, which can contribute to burnout (Cumming & Wong, 2019, p.275). The practice vignette below explores the emotional impact of working with children and families facing adversity.

 Practice vignette

Collette is a young practitioner who has recently started working in a Pupil Referral Unit (PRU). As part of her responsibilities, she undertakes home visits to a family whose son, Carl attends the unit. Carl is usually brought to the PRU by his older sister, often wearing clothes that look as if they have been slept in and is usually unwashed and hungry.

The home visit is a shocking experience for Collette. She discovers that Carl's mother is living with another women who also has several children. They both work as sex workers during the night, usually with one of the women staying at home to look after the children, but occasionally both working at the same time. There are no home comforts; the children sleep on dirty mattresses; the floor and cupboards are bare and there is an air of hopelessness permeating the house behind the boarded up front door. The family has two dogs who are locked in the kitchen when Collette visits, but bark and throw themselves against the door continually.

Carl's mother, Lexi, is wary of Collette at first, but over time she comes to see Collette as a confidant, sharing her difficult experiences at school when she was young and the abuse she suffered from a family friend. Collette starts to keep an eye out for items to give to Lexi, such as curtains for the children's bedroom so they can sleep better. She helps Lexi apply to a charity for beds and a cooker.

When the six-week holiday arrives, Collette no longer sees Carl or Lexi, yet she cannot get them out of her mind. She worries how Carl and his siblings are coping and finds herself crying for no reason. She wakes in the night wondering if she could have done more to help. Collette passes Carl's home on her way to the supermarket and tries to see how things are going as she drives past, but it just makes her more depressed and feel more tearful and anxious.

Eventually, Collette discusses this with her supervisor and recognises that she may be struggling with burnout. They put some boundaries and strategies in place, including driving a different way to the supermarket, finding ways to boost her mood, such as listening to music with happy memories and taking time to rest. Her supervisor reassures her that she went beyond what would be expected of a practitioner and that she must not assume a burden of responsibility for the family.

Critical question

- How can Collette take positive actions to support her own wellbeing, following this experience, and how can her supervisor best support her?

Stress

Stress is the neurological and psychological change that occurs in our bodies when we feel threatened. This may be from external sources, such as family expectations or lack of time, or internal sources, such as self-criticism, or a loss of control (Nagoski & Nagoski, 2020). We frequently use the word 'stressed' to express how we are feeling, but it is an umbrella term encompassing a range of underlying issues that we cannot adequately deal with. When we pinpoint the cause of stress, we can take steps to deal with the issue; if not, we risk being unable to progress (Nagoski & Nagoski, 2020) and, the body remains in a fight or flight state, necessary for emergencies, but the increased blood pressure exacerbates the risk of serious disease if experienced continually (Nagoski & Nagoski, 2020).

According to the Health and Safety Executive (n.d.) stress at work centres around six main areas:

- The job is too demanding
- Lack of control
- Lack of support
- Poor relationships
- Not fully understanding the role
- Not being part of changes.

Other contributors to low wellbeing

Another risk for those involved in emotional labour is navigating the intersection of professional love and the love we have for our own family (Page & Elfer, 2013). In addition, caring for several children at once requires constant negotiation of our attention distribution, being alert to children's individual cues (de Schipper *et al.*, 2006), particularly intense when working with pre-verbal and non-speaking children (de Schipper *et al.*, 2006).

Much work with trauma-experienced children and families is provided by Third Sector organisations, funded through project grants, often for fixed periods. When the funding dries up there is the stress of applying for further grants and, if successful, complying with potentially different regulations (Cumming & Wong, 2019). This may also affect pay and conditions, and although practitioners do not work with children and families to become rich, a sense of 'financial wellbeing', feeling content that you have sufficient means to meet your current financial obligations and future aspirations (Aubrey *et al.*, 2022) is a significant factor in overall wellbeing. Many practitioners consider themselves not only underpaid but ignored by policy makers, also contributing to low wellbeing (Solvason & Webb, 2023).

A hectic schedule and constant demands when working at full capacity will cause stress and exhaustion. We should be concerned, however, when any action, for example, resting, taking vitamins or going on holiday, does not restore our equilibrium (Institute for Quality and Efficiency in Health Care, 2020).

The three Ps

Using the social pedagogy concept of the three Ps (Kaska, 2015) can ensure that our professional, personal and private selves are borne in mind when working with children and families (see Chapters 4 and 5 for more on the three Ps). Although it is essential that we use the warmth of our personalities to establish and maintain trusting relationships (personal) it is equally important to maintain a professional boundary. Being friendly is to be encouraged but this should not develop into inappropriate friendships where we may reveal an aspect of our lives that ought to remain private. To protect our wellbeing, we must discipline ourselves not to assume the challenges of children and families as if they were our own. Wallowing in the pain felt by trauma-experienced children does not help them or you and delineating between the professional, personal and private is essential. If not, we may experience poor wellbeing and even compassion fatigue, burnout and stress "not because we do not care, but because we have been caring too much for too long" (Moxley, 2022, p.8).

Critical questions

- Can you identify with any of these issues?
- Can you talk to a leader in your workplace about it?
- Do you recognise any symptoms in anyone you work with?
- Who do you work with who seems to manage their stress? What strategies do they employ?

Why we need to address wellbeing at work

As have discussed, low wellbeing at work can impact negatively on our health, relationships and overall wellbeing. On the other hand, work can be therapeutic, warding off the adverse effects of being unemployed (Waddell & Burton, 2006). When we see that we matter and are making a difference to children's lives, this contributes to our wellbeing.

Better performance and outcomes

When practitioners have high wellbeing studies have shown that their interactions with children are of a higher quality, offering opportunities to practise and extend skills (Carnahan et.al., 2009), which is positively linked to children's achievement (McWilliam & Bailey, 1995). The nature of children's interactions with practitioners also has long-term significance for how they manage emotional experiences, communicate feelings effectively, learn how to cope with frustrating situations (Bailey, 2013, p.132) and develop resilience (Bouillet et al., 2014). When practitioners model these traits, children's self-efficacy, responsibility (Arastaman & Balci, 2013) and educational success is supported (Denham et al., 2012). They are more likely to become well-adjusted adults with good mental health and wellbeing (Khanlou & Wray, 2014).

Co-regulation

As we understand more about how children develop positive behaviour, the focus shifts from taking a behaviourist, behaviour management approach, i.e., using rewards and sanctions to condition children into compliance, to self-regulation (Robson & Zachariou, 2022). Shanker (2017) proposed that when children are not in a calm and focused state they are unable to regulate their behaviour, and practitioners and others should assist (co-regulation) by de-escalating their stress and restoring them to a calm state. Robson and Zachariou (2022) use the analogy of learning to ride a bike to illustrate the concept of co-regulation and self-regulation. The adult supports and guides the child, gradually withdrawing support until they can do it alone.

If the adult has not mastered this skill themselves, however, shouting at the child for being unable to do it, or humiliates them when they wobble, the child is unlikely to be motivated to persist or master the skills they need. Similarly, to support children's self-regulation we must first be able to self-regulate ourselves (Moxley, 2022). This means taking responsibility for how our emotions can affect workplace environments and being good role models for children and other practitioners. Attending to our own wellbeing, therefore, is crucial for having the emotional energy to co-regulate with children (Moxley, 2022), particularly as children's challenging behaviour is itself a source of stress (Friedman-Krauss et al., 2013).

What can be done

Wellbeing at work is affected by many interrelated factors and attempts to improve it must take this into account. Although individuals can take action to enhance their wellbeing, employing organisations also have a responsibility to develop support systems that contribute to a culture of wellbeing at work (Corr et al., 2015).

The employers' responsibility

Many employers do pay attention to employee wellbeing (Stringer, 2023). We live in a tick box culture, however, and there is a danger that this is reduced to one-off, tokenistic gestures rather than an overarching commitment to changing organisational culture, policy and procedures and, ultimately, actions. A few lead practitioners have shared with Nicola and Alison some of the things they do to show that they care about staff wellbeing. These include:

- Mindful colouring books in staff areas
- Giving staff members the day off on their birthday
- Sending flowers for work anniversaries
- Providing lunch (usually eaten with the children)
- Giving gift baskets with personal care items
- Notice boards promoting wellbeing.

In a supportive environment where the whole team contributes to a nurturing environment, these gestures will only increase morale. If, however, there is incongruence between what is said and what is done, if some people seem to 'get away' with doing less or if policies and procedures are not applied with equity (for example, expectations of attendance at staff meetings, or when time off can be taken), these gestures are seen as empty and will not make up for poor employee performance management, indifference and low wellbeing (Stringer, 2023).

 Case study: primary school teacher Phoebe Burton

Phoebe Burton was one of Nicola and Alison's students who studied for an Early Childhood degree. She became interested in how to support children's self-regulation because she knew that she would encounter children struggling with stress, from the death of a family member to being unable to zip up their coat. Phoebe decided to make self-regulation the subject of her dissertation. She is now a qualified primary school teacher working in an area of deprivation. Here Phoebe reflects on the findings of her dissertation.

> The staff team at the kindergarten where I conducted my research were very nurturing, both towards me and the children and families who attended. They had a policy of

co-regulation rather than behaviour management and I was keen to learn how they managed to implement this so successfully. I had been attending the setting for a few months but was still surprised at what came out during the data gathering.

"Responding thoughtfully can only happen if you're feeling OK," revealed one practitioner, sharing that they practise 'mindfulness' to enable them to be mindfully in the moment with the child because "this allows you to be responsive instead of reactive". However, practitioners also shared that when co-regulating with a child "it can feel like all your ability to regulate is given to them (the child)"; another stated, "it can get hard" and "it can be exhausting"; "you cannot fight fire with fire, to regulate a child in a crisis the adult must first be calm – self-care is vital".

I began to appreciate how important a shared commitment to wellbeing is for enabling practitioners to maintain a high level of concentration and the giving of themselves. When they were in danger of feeling overwhelmed and dysregulated, they felt safe to "tap out", "swap with another practitioner" or "take a 5-minute break".

One way the setting owners showed that practitioner wellbeing was of priority was that only one member of staff worked full time because, as they explained, "this job, done well, is exhausting". They also invested in cultivating knowledgeable practitioners and understood that to perform at their best they needed time to rest and "re-charge". The owners would put together 'nurture packages' for the staff that contained items such as supplements, books and self-care products.

The vital connection between practitioner wellbeing and co-regulation with children was a key finding of my study. I began it assuming I would find strategies for practice to promote children's self-regulation, however it has become much more personal and meaningful to me. As practitioners we place high importance on children's wellbeing, however, to be effective, we must be mentally, physically and emotionally strong enough to support this, recognise when we are not and take time out to recuperate.

This had a positive impact on me when I qualified as a primary school teacher. I understand the importance looking after my own wellbeing has for the children, and I try to make this a priority. And yet, I also need to find effective ways of doing this when time is in very short supply.

I hope to be a leader of practice someday and practitioner wellbeing is something I will prioritise. Ensuring practitioners know they are cared for and appreciated, as well as offering 'real-life' strategies to improve mental health and wellbeing, rather than superficial or 'tick box' activities, will play a big part in my approach.

Critical questions

1. How did the practitioners make wellbeing and self-care part of the setting culture?
2. How did the owners go beyond a tick box approach to wellbeing?
3. What challenge did Phoebe still need to resolve? Can you offer any suggestions to resolve her difficulty?

Supporting Children's Mental Health and Wellbeing

Accessing supervision

When working with children and families experiencing difficulties, we may worry both about them and whether some aspect of support was overlooked. This can feel like "a heavy bag that we just can't put down" (Stephen & Nettleton, 2022, p.53) and accessing good-quality supervision can help lighten our load. Supervision is a requirement in many professions and involves practitioners meeting regularly with a trained supervisor to discuss safeguarding concerns, and other professional issues, offering "space to make sense of our own feelings through the mind of another" (Stephen & Nettleton, 2022, p.57). Talking through concerns in a structured way can help us process experiences and restore our emotional equilibrium, which is essential for our continuing engagement at work (Stephen & Nettleton, 2022, p.57).

Boundaries and strategies

Making sure you put in appropriate boundaries to maintain a good work/life balance is an ongoing challenge but doing so signals to others that you value yourself and encourages them to do the same, contributing to a culture of healthy wellbeing.

> **REFLECTIVE TASK**
>
> Table 11.1 shows some examples of boundaries and strategies. Can you complete the rationale? The first one has been completed as an example.

Table 11.1 Boundaries, strategies and rationale for improved wellbeing

Boundary or strategy	Rationale
Be aware of what foods you eat. Foods with a low GI (glycaemic index) enable the body to maintain a steady condition, e.g., lentils, beans, wholegrain cereal, etc.	Food can significantly affect our mood and stress levels. Highly processed food, i.e., high in salt and fat, raises cortisol levels and adrenaline. We get a sugar high with an accompanying crash, resulting in more sugar cravings.
Drink water to hydrate	
Make changes in your diet slowly	
Make time to eat	
Start and finish work on time	
Only send and read work texts and emails during working hours (this means taking them off your phone)	
Put activities that you enjoy doing in your diary, e.g., exercising, reading, crafting, choir or playing on a games console	
Talk to friends, have a good laugh	
Appreciate the outdoors	
Practise self-compassion	
Journal regularly	
Take opportunities for training and Continuing Professional Development	
Concentrate on what you can control	

Supporting our own wellbeing 157

Positive self-talk and affirmations

There is tremendous power in thoughts, and they have a huge influence on the type of person we develop into. Sometimes we can get into a destructive cycle of thinking that influences how we feel, behave and imagine others perceive us. This can affect our wellbeing, so noticing when this happens and taking action to reverse the cycle is important (Moxley, 2022). Having some simple, rehearsed affirmative statements ready when you start to feel overwhelmed can be empowering for regaining inner calm and boost your mood.

Some examples include:

- What would I say to a friend in this situation?
- Will this matter in five years?
- This is not about me, I am taking this personally.
- I am doing the best I can.
- I'd rather not have to deal with this, but I can manage it.

Over time you will gather your own affirmations, and using them as a mental health first aid support can lower immediate anxiety.

Working with a mental health condition

In the past, there was a stigma around mental health resulting in professionals being wary of being open about their own. We may think that our professional role requires us to be strong and that we must be perfectly emotionally stable to avoid the negative judgement of others. We are not robots, however, and everyone experiences the highs and lows of life, some of which will affect our mental health (Stephen & Nettleton, 2022). Moxley (2022, p.15) suggests that we should "dispel issues of ableism in our understanding of well-being" and challenge the assumption that having a mental health diagnosis will result in lower effectiveness when "the reality is ... that many of us have a diagnosis and may always live with a mental illness" (Moxley, 2022, p.15). This does not preclude anyone from living a productive and happy life and may be a strength for empathetic practice (Stephen & Nettleton, 2022).

Conclusion

This chapter considered the importance of safeguarding practitioner wellbeing, a risk factor when working with children and families experiencing difficulties. There are many reasons why those engaging in emotional labour may experience low wellbeing, activated by continuous emotional attunement to children's needs. Without careful management this can result in compassion fatigue, burnout and stress. There is evidence that practitioner wellbeing impacts on children's outcomes, both cognitively and emotionally and therefore it should be prioritised by employers and practitioners in a symbiotic way. We should remember that many practitioners have experienced episodes of low wellbeing and poor mental health but that this should not be a barrier to working with children and families, in fact it may give them an empathetic edge.

Supporting our own wellbeing: key points

- 'Mental health' and 'wellbeing' are often used interchangeably but are different.
- Wellbeing is not fixed, but everyone has a 'set point' of wellbeing.
- Physical, mental, emotional, social and spiritual wellbeing are all interconnected.
- Work-related wellbeing plays a significant role in our overall life satisfaction.
- Working with children and families can be emotionally draining, potentially resulting in vicarious trauma.
- Compassion fatigue, burnout, stress and other factors contributes to low wellbeing.
- Applying the social pedagogy concept of the three Ps (Kaska, 2015) may be helpful in avoiding giving too much of ourselves.
- Children achieve better outcomes when practitioners have high wellbeing.
- To support children's self-regulation skills practitioners must be able to self-regulate themselves (Moxley, 2022).
- Employers have a responsibility to ensure that the work culture supports worker wellbeing. This extends beyond one-off gestures.
- Practitioners can take steps to support their own wellbeing, including accessing supervision, establishing boundaries and strategies, engaging in positive self-talk and affirmations.
- Working with a mental health condition does not preclude us from working effectively with children and families and may be a strength.

ADDITIONAL RESOURCES

- Beaumont, E. and Irons, C. (2017) *The compassionate mind workbook: a step-by-step guide to developing your compassionate self*. London: Robinson.

A thought-provoking book that considers that the way the brain works can result in anxious thoughts and physiological symptoms such as nausea, increased heartrate and anger. It proposes taking a deliberate, compassionate approach and applying it to ourselves. Written in an accessible style, there are explanations of how our brains work, why we respond the way we do and exercises to help break anxiety loops.

- The Wellness Recovery Action Plan (WRAP). Available at: file:///C:/Users/admin/Downloads/WRAP_Book_A4.pdf.

WRAP is a tool to help you through difficult times and plan a positive future. The link above takes you to a workbook of exercises to guide your wellbeing journey.

References

Arastaman, G. and Balci, A. (2013) Investigation of high school students' resiliency perception in terms of some variables. *Educational Science: Theory & Practice*, 13(2), pp. 922-928.

Aubrey, M., Morin, A.J.S., Fernet, C. and Carbonneau, N. (2022) Financial wellbeing: capturing an elusive construct with an optimized measure. *Frontiers in Psychology*, 13(935284), pp. 1-18. doi: 10.3389/fpsyg.2022.935284.

Bailey, C.S., Zinsser, K.M., Curby, T.W., Denham, S.A. and Bassett, H.H. (2013) Consistently emotionally supportive preschool teachers and children's social-emotional learning in the classroom: implications for center directors and teachers. *Health Education*, 16(2), pp. 131-137. doi: 10.1108/HE-11-2013-0062.

Bloechliger, O.R. and Bauer, G.F. (2016) Demands and job resources in the childcare workforce: Swiss lead teachers and assistant teacher assessments. *Early Education and Development*, 27(7), pp. 1040-1059.

Bouillet, D., Ivanec, P.T. and Miljević-Riđički, R. (2014) Preschool teachers' resilience and their readiness for building children's resilience. *Health Education*, 114(6), pp. 435-450. doi: 10.1108/HE-11-2013-0062.

Bradford, H. (2012) *The wellbeing of children under three*. London. Routledge.

Bullough, R.V. and Hall-Kenyon, K.M. (2018) *Preschool teachers' lives and work: stories and studies from the field*. New York: Routledge.

Carnahan, C., Musti-Rao, S. and Bailey, J. (2009). Promoting active engagement in small group learning experiences for students with autism and significant learning needs. *Education and Treatment of Children*, 32(1), pp. 37-61. Available at: www.jstor.org/stable/42900006.

Corr, L., Cook, K., LaMontagne, A.D., Waters, E. and Davis, E. (2015) Associations between Australian early childhood educators' mental health and working conditions. *Australasian Journal of Early Childhood*, 40(3), pp. 69-78.

Cumming, T. and Wong, S. (2019) Towards a holistic conceptualisation of early childhood educators' work-related wellbeing. *Contemporary Issues in Early Childhood*, 20(3), pp. 265-281. doi: https://doi.org/10.1177/1463949118772573.

Cummins, R.A., Ning, L., Stokes, M. and Wooden, M. (2014) A demonstration of set-points for subjective wellbeing. *Journal of Happiness Studies*, 15(1), pp. 183-206.

Denham, S., Bassett, H. and Zinsser, K. (2012) Early childhood teachers as socializers of young children's emotional competence. *Early Childhood Education Journal*, 40(3), pp. 137-143. doi: 10.1007/s10643-012-0504-2.

de Schipper, E.J., Riksen-Walraven, J.M. and Geurts, S.A. (2006) Effects of child-caregiver ratio on the interactions between caregivers and children in child-care centers: an experimental study, *Child Development*, 77(4), pp. 861-874. doi: 10.1111/j.1467-8624.2006.00907. x.

Dodge, R., Daly, A.P., Huyton, J. and Sanders, L.D. (2012) The challenge of defining wellbeing. *International Journal of Wellbeing*, 2(3), pp. 222-235.

Ettema, D. and Schekkerman, M. (2016) How do spatial characteristics influence wellbeing and mental health? Comparing the effect of objective and subjective characteristics at different spatial scales. *Travel Behaviour and Society* 5(September), 56-67. doi: https://doi.org/10.1016/j.tbs.2015.11.001.

Freudenberger, H. (1975) The staff burn out syndrome in alternative institutions, *Psychotherapy: Theory, Research and Practice* (12), pp. 73-82.

Friedman-Krauss, A.H., Raver, C.C., Neuspiel, J.M. and Kinsel, J. (2013) Child behavior problems, teacher executive functions, and teacher stress in head start classrooms. *Early Education and Development*, 25(5), pp. 681-702. doi: https://doi.org/10.1080/10409289.2013.825190.

Gillett-Swan, J.K. and Sargeant, J. (2015) Wellbeing as a process of accrual: beyond subjectivity and beyond the moment. *Social Indicators Research*, 121(1), pp. 135-148. doi: 10.1007/s11205-014-0634-6.

Health and Safety Executive (n.d.) *Work-related stress and how to manage it*. Available at: https://www.hse.gov.uk/stress/causes.htm (Accessed 23 September 2024).

Hochschild, A.R. (1983) *The managed heart*. Berkeley, CA: University of California Press.

Institute for Quality and Efficiency in Health Care (2020) *What is burnout?* Available at: https://www.ncbi.nlm.nih.gov/books/NBK279286 (Accessed 23 September 2024).

Kaska (2015). *Social pedagogy, an invitation*. London, Jacaranda Development.

Khanlou, N. and Wray, R. (2014) A whole community approach toward child and youth resilience promotion: a review of resilience literature. *International Journal of Mental Health Addiction*, 12(1), pp. 64-79.

Kusma, B., Groneberg, D.A., Mache, S. and Nienhaus, A. (2012) Determinants of day care teachers' job satisfaction. *Central European Journal of Public Health*, 20(3), pp. 191–198.

McWilliam, R.A., Trivette, C.M. and Dunst, C.J. (1985) Behavior engagement as a measure of the efficacy of early intervention. *Analysis and Intervention in Developmental Disabilities*, 5(1–2), pp. 59–71.

Moxley, K. (2022) *A guide to mental health for early years educators: putting wellbeing at the heart of your philosophy and practice*. 1st edn. London: Routledge.

Nagoski, E. and Nagoski, A. (2020) *Burnout: solve your stress cycle*. London: Vermillion.

Nelinger, A., Album, J., Haynes, A. and Rosan, C. (2021) Their challenges are our challenges: a summary report of the experiences facing nursery workers in the UK in 2020. Anna Freud Centre for Children and Families. Available at: https://d1uw1dikibnh8j.cloudfront.net/media/13013/their-challenges-are-our-challenges-survey-report.pdf (Accessed 20 September 2024).

Organisation for Economic Co-operation and Development (OECD) (2022) Promoting health and wellbeing at work: policy and practices, *OECD Health Policy Studies*. Paris: OECD Publishing. Available at: file:///C:/Users/admin/Downloads/e179b2a5-en.pdf (Accessed 19 September 2024).

Page, J. and Elfer, P. (2013) The emotional complexity of attachment interactions in nursery, *European Early Childhood Education Research Journal*, 21(4), pp. 553–567.

Parker, C. (2020). Creative mentoring: a creative response to promote learning and wellbeing with children in care. A service developed by Derbyshire County Council's Virtual School. *International Journal of Social Pedagogy*, 9(1), pp. 1–15. doi: https://doi.org/10.14324/111.444.ijsp.2020.v9.x.005.

Robson, S. and Zachariou, A. (2022) *Self-regulation in the early years*. London: Sage.

Royer, N. and Moreau, C. (2015) A survey of Canadian early childhood educators' psychological wellbeing at work. *Early Childhood Education Journal*, 44(2), pp. 135–146. doi: 10.1007/ s10643-015-0696-3.

Shanker, S. (2017). What you need to know. Self-regulation: the early years. The MEHRIT Centre. Available at: https://self-reg.ca/wp-content/uploads/2021/05/infosheet_The-Early-Years.pdf (Accessed 26 September 2024).

Simmons, L.A. and Wright, O. (2023) Vicarious trauma, compassion fatigue and burnout: tools for EMDR therapists. EMDR Therapy Quarterly. Available at: https://etq.emdrassociation.org.uk/2023/10/17/vicarious-trauma-compassion-fatigue-and-burnout-tools-for-emdr-therapists (Accessed 20 September 2024).

Solvason, C. and Webb, R. (eds.) (2023) *Exploring and celebrating the early childhood practitioner: an interrogation of pedagogy, professionalism and practice*. Abingdon: Routledge.

Stephen, R. and Nettleton, R. (2022) Professional practice and practitioner wellbeing, in Burrows, P. and Cowie, J. (eds.) *Health visiting, specialist community public health nursing*. 3rd edn. London: Elsevier Health Sciences.

Stringer, H. (2023) *Worker wellbeing is in demand as organizational culture shifts*. American Psychological Association. Available at: https://www.apa.org/monitor/2023/01/trends-worker-wellbeing (Accessed 26 September 2024).

Waddell, G. and Burton, A.K. (2006) *Is work good for your health and wellbeing?* The Stationary Office. Available at: https://cardinal-management.co.uk/wp-content/uploads/2016/04/Burton-Waddell-is-work-good-for-you.pdf (Accessed 26 September 2024).

World Health Organization (2022) *Mental health factsheet*. Available at: https://www.who.int/news-room/fact-sheets/detail/mental-health-strengthening-our-response (Accessed 19 September 2014).

World Health Organization (n.d.) Constitution of the World Health Organization. Available at: https://www.who.int/about/governance/constitution (Accessed 19 September 2024).

12
Bringing it all together and next steps

Introduction

This book has explored many of the issues affecting children and families today. We recognise that in our post pandemic world, the future is more uncertain than ever before, and this, combined with other factors such as social media, can have negative impacts on children and young people's wellbeing. It is against this challenging background that this book is situated. We have woven together a narrative that highlights the profound difference that intentional, compassionate interventions delivered by attuned and trustworthy practitioners can make to the lives of children and families. Through the lenses of various therapeutic approaches, we have explored how bespoke and tailored support can foster resilience, healing and growth in the face of life's multiple challenges. This chapter provides a summary of the messages of the book and considers the vital role of the practitioner in delivering high-quality therapeutic interventions in the context of strong and trustful relationships. Finally, we provide an opportunity for readers to reflect upon their own practice and to identify areas where the messages of the book can provide inspiration for action planning to support children and families.

Therapeutic approaches, a summary

Chapter 1 began by examining a range of possible factors that have led to the increase in mental health issues among children and young people, contextualised within the current social, cultural and political landscape. In this first chapter we defined what we mean by a therapeutic approach, with a case study from a therapeutic foster carer used as illustration. We defined and outlined three possible approaches to therapeutic work (psychodynamic, person-centred and cognitive) before exploring the merits of an integrative approach. We postulated that there is a growing need for practitioners to be upskilled in therapeutic approaches when supporting children and families. In highlighting the long-term implications of childhood adversity, we suggested that doing nothing was not an option. Similarly, we explored the implications of doing the wrong things, including the importance of not overreaching our roles and ensuring we seek specialist input where it is appropriate.

In Chapter 2 we considered the critical issue of childhood adversity. The chapter began with a discussion of the definitions of adversity, drawing on previous research which highlighted both the breadth and depth of scale and difficulty, before adding our own dimension – the longevity of the adversity. The chapter explored the diverse experiences of adversity (for example, bereavement and loss, marginalisation, discrimination, poverty, mental health issues, addiction, homelessness, displacement and racism) which may impact on children's lives. We then considered the effects of such adversity on children's emotional wellbeing, behaviour and relationships. Government agendas on adverse childhood experiences (ACEs) were also critically considered. We stressed the potential of applying a strength-based approach, and considered the importance of resilience and hope, especially within difficult experiences and circumstances. The case study for this chapter focused on the experience of Layla (a child constructed from the practice experience of a practitioner in an alternative provision setting), where we can see that the adversity Layla faced has impacted on all aspects of her life and relationships.

Chapter 3 began by exploring attachment and the need for sensitive and attuned relationships. We stressed that practitioners need to be mindful of the phenomenon of attachment sabotaging, and we explored how to read and re-frame challenging behaviour as communication. Key principles of the successful Circles of Security programme were outlined, including addressing when adults themselves have an unresolved insecure attachment; a case study was included as an example of a family-supported intervention. The chapter explored the importance of going beyond an instrumental key person approach, by seeing the whole child, with the concept of life world orientation used as a theoretical framework. We then considered how we can elevate our practice using Pestalozzi's Head, Heart and Hands as a tool to truly focus on holistic wellbeing. We explored how we can foster an emotionally safe and enabling environment that meets children's psychological needs.

Chapter 4 discussed some of the benefits of play, particularly for trauma-experienced children. The chapter began by exploring how play in general supports children's development, particularly physical, mental and cognitive development. We then focused on risky play and its role in building resilience and self-determined behaviour. The conceptual model of the Learning Zone provided a useful theoretical framework to underpin the chapter. Next, we examined how play therapy delivered by clinically trained play therapists can help children to process trauma; a case study of play therapy in a hospital was used to illustrate this. We explored general guidance about the adoption of the therapeutic, play-based approach PACE, which can be used by all practitioners. A play-based emotional coaching scenario demonstrating how fostering meaningful relationships can be taught to children through play was critically examined. The chapter concluded with some practical ideas for play with therapeutic elements to try out in practice.

Chapter 5 examined the power of creativity and its role in supporting those who have experienced trauma and adversity. The chapter began by defining creativity and outlining its value for child development. We then presented evidence of how art and music can be a vehicle for fostering attachment, contributing to a sense of belonging and esteem. Self-determination theory, the three basic psychological needs and the link to creativity were critically explored. We also considered the power of flow in creativity for increasing wellbeing. The chapter proceeded to consider how drama can foster resilience and an internal locus of control. We explored the potential of artistic activities as a vehicle for processing and healing after mild trauma with some pointers for success, stressing the importance of building positive relationships with children and families in all therapeutic work. The conceptual model

Bringing it all together and next steps 163

of the three Ps and the use of Common Third activities were suggested as tools to ensure appropriate relationships can develop. We considered what action to take when things go wrong and suggested that rushing children through their trauma processing is mistaken. A case study from a person-centred therapist was used to illustrate the points discussed throughout the chapter.

Chapter 6 examined the measurable health and developmental benefits of being outdoors, including those related to risky play outdoors. A case study from a Forest School setting demonstrated the power of the outdoors in the process of healing. This led to the consideration of more holistic benefits, such as the use of outdoors as a retreat, and how a sense of place can offer a secure attachment similar to the care-giver bond. The chapter explored Attention Restoration Theory and outlined the four criteria that make an environment restorative, concluding that the natural world has the potential to meet all these measures. We detailed how this is of particular interest to those working in the fields of ADHD, mental fatigue and stress recovery. The chapter also invited us, however, to explore more deeply an over-simplified discourse of childhood and the accessibility of the outdoors for all. Finally, we called on practitioners to promote the special benefits of the great outdoors before these are lost.

Chapter 7 focused on mindfulness as a helpful tool for self-regulation and countering anxiety. The evidence base for this expanding area of practice was critically explored, with a focus on its benefits and how mindful approaches can be nurtured and developed by attuned practitioners. The chapter explored how a mindful approach can allow individuals, especially those who have experienced trauma, to remain in the moment, moving beyond the stresses of past and future. We argued that focusing on being in the present can heighten awareness of thoughts, feelings and the world around us, leading to increased emotional wellbeing. The chapter outlined a range of mindfulness techniques and suggested activities that can help children acquire a disposition of mindfulness, using skills which, once learned, can be self-administered to alleviate stress. The mind–body connection was explored with reference to the benefits of yoga and progressive muscle relaxation. The case study for this chapter was provided by a dance psychotherapist who explored how dance can help us attune to and express our inner thoughts and feelings. She introduced us to the term 'bodyfulness', a practice which helps us move beyond awareness and into action. This can be particularly helpful for children who can gain benefits of meaning making and letting go, through moving their bodies in a creative and playful way.

Chapter 8 explored the contributions of talking therapies to children's wellbeing. Whilst we recognised that there are a range of talking therapies including psychotherapy, counselling and family group conferencing, the chapter recognised that these require registration with regulatory bodies and extensive additional training to administer them. Hence the chapter focused strongly on cognitive approaches to therapy. Cognitive behavioural therapy (CBT) and dialectical behaviour therapy (DBT) are critically explored in relation to their relative benefits and the challenges associated with their delivery. We suggested that whilst these approaches need to be delivered by trained and qualified therapists, there are useful techniques that can be applied more generically to help children and young people. The chapter is underpinned by the conceptual model of the CBT vicious cycle, which explores the interconnection and self-perpetuating nature of thoughts, feelings and behaviours. The case study, which consisted of a conversation with two practitioners who work in an intensive support service for care-experienced children and their families, provided an insight into the importance of attuned responsiveness, relationship building and self-care when working therapeutically with others. The chapter also considered the importance of Theory of Mind (ToM) and mentalising as a first step towards the use of cognitive approaches, recognising that prior to any CBT intervention, the individual must be able to recognise a thought, to know how it differs from a feeling and to appreciate that others may think differently.

Chapter 9 considered how stories (both our own stories and the stories of others) can be used to support wellbeing. We considered how metaphors, stories and fables can become tools of therapeutic intervention, as they provide a vehicle for children to express their thoughts and feelings, and in doing so gain deeper understandings of themselves and their world. We considered how creating and telling stories can help children to develop a personal voice, expressing their own unique ways of thinking, feeling and being. We explored a range of diverse ways of supporting storytelling, including the use of puppetry, props and digital media.

The chapter then introduced the concept of bibliotherapy, a process by which stories allow children to explore and understand prominent issues affecting their lives through story books and other written materials. We postulated that interpreting stories is an ever-changing process to which children bring their own needs and experiences. Since children (especially those who have experienced trauma) often have difficulty identifying and communicating their feelings, we argued that stories can serve to facilitate open discussion and self-understanding.

The case study for this chapter featured children's author, Sue Barrow, who explained how books can help children to understand difficult societal issues. Sue drew examples from her own work *Sold*, a young adult book based around trafficking and modern-day slavery, and *Keeping Secrets*, a story about adoption, focusing on the emotions and experiences of the young person at the centre of the story. This case study provided useful insights into the value of stories for promoting voice, understanding and healing. Finally, the chapter considered the value of writing as a tool for critical reflection and encouraged readers to engage in their own writing adventures to support personal development and enhance practice.

Chapter 10 considered the important role of the practitioner in supporting therapeutic work with children and families. We considered what it means to be an attuned practitioner and explored the critical area of active listening. Readers were challenged to consider their own knowledge, skills and dispositions in relation to supporting children's holistic wellbeing. We also considered the importance of unconditional positive regard (UPR) and listening without judgement. The social pedagogy tenet of Head, Heart and Hands was critically explored. The chapter included two practice vignettes designed to illustrate how attunement and UPR are manifested in practice. The case study for this chapter was linked to the one provided in Chapter 2 and we considered what an attuned approach to supporting Layla could look like and the role of the practitioner within that. The chapter concluded with a consideration of the importance of intentionally setting the scene for attunement by creating a conducive physical and emotional environment in which attunement can happen.

Bringing it all together and next steps 165

Continuing our focus on the individual practitioner, Chapter 11 clarified what is meant by wellbeing, including how it differs from mental health, how it is unique to everyone and incorporates physical, mental, emotional, social and spiritual aspects. The chapter explored how work-related wellbeing contributes to overall wellbeing and why those who work with children and families are particularly prone to wellbeing depletion. The blurred line between our professional and personal self, the cost of emotional attunement, compassion fatigue, burnout and stress were all considered in depth. The three Ps were discussed as a way of safeguarding our core self. The chapter went on to consider the reasons why work-related wellbeing should be addressed, including the positive impact it has on children's academic performance and self-regulation skills. Finally, the chapter invited us to review both the employer's and the practitioner's responsibility to foster wellbeing and concluded by addressing the issue of working while living with a mental health condition.

REFLECTIVE TASK

It is now timely to encourage practitioners to reflect on and apply the therapeutic approaches from the book to their own practice with children and families. The following reflective activity encourages you to consider each chapter in turn and to draw together the main points of your learning before identifying how you might take this learning forward. You may wish to complete Table 12.1 and keep it as a record of your learning and planned actions. The first section has been completed for you as an example.

Some final thoughts

As we close this exploration of therapeutic approaches to supporting children and families, it is evident that no single approach holds all the answers. The true strength of therapeutic work lies in its bespoke nature and its adaptability and responsiveness to the unique needs of each child and family. Within this book we have explored a range of evidence-based interventions. However, whether using creative approaches, mindfulness or the structured skills of CBT, the core message remains that connection, understanding and commitment to positive change are the cornerstones of effective support. Its success depends as much on *how we are* with families as *what we do* alongside them. Hence, our ways of being and interacting become interventions in their own right, as we model anti-oppressive, person-centred, democratic and respectful interventions that embody hope and the potential for positive change. In the hands of dedicated practitioners, these dispositions and approaches become powerful tools for releasing the potential within each child and family to navigate their own journeys with greater ease. Hence, our aspiration is for this book to serve as a conversation starter, a resource and, hopefully, a tiny grain of inspiration reminding us that through our collective efforts we can create a world where children and families feel seen, supported and empowered to flourish.

Table 12.1 Personal action plan based on learning from each chapter

Chapter	Main points of personal learning	How this aligns with my practice	My actions	Any further reflections
Chapter 1: An introduction to working therapeutically with children and families	The three basic approaches to working therapeutically.	My practice implicitly aligns with all the approaches, but I haven't considered this consciously.	Be aware of each approach and which is the best one to take with children and families.	Share my thoughts with other practitioners to foster a whole team approach.
Chapter 2: Understanding adversity				
Chapter 3: Supporting the holistic needs of children and families				
Chapter 4: The importance of play				
Chapter 5: The role of creativity in supporting those who have experienced adversity				
Chapter 6: The great outdoors				
Chapter 7: A mindful approach				
Chapter 8: Talking therapies				
Chapter 9: The power of stories				
Chapter 10: The attuned practitioner				
Chapter 11: Supporting our own wellbeing.				
Chapter 12: Bringing it all together and next steps				

Index

acceptance 25, 54, 108
acceptance and commitment therapy (ACT) 109
active listening 135, 137
ADHD 7, 53, 83-84, 121
adult as containers 71
adverse childhood experiences 4, 18-19, 53; criticism of 19
adversity 17-20
Ainsworth, M. 32, 50, 54, 82
amygdala 23, 33
anxiety 6-7, 54, 68, 90-94, 97, 104-105, 107-108, 137; and COVID-19 4; in PTSD 22; and insecure attachment 33-34; and self-determination theory 42-43
art therapy 64, 68
attachment: adult insecure 36; attention seeking verses attachment needing 35; and attunement 135, 148; definition and categories 32-33; and key person 38; to place 82; and play 50; sabotaging 34; see also creativity and early attachment
attention restoration theory 82-83
attunement 133; and attachment theory 135; emotional cost of 148
austerity 4-5
avenues of hope 68

behavioural activation 105
behaviour as communication 34-35, 137
bereavement 33, 162
bibliotherapy 12-121
body 23, 151, 163
'bodyfulness' 163
body language 134

body scan 93
boundaries 108, 144; professional boundaries 149
Bourdieu see cultural capital
Bowlby, J. 32, 35, 82
brain 19, 23-25, 50
breathing 90; breathing exercises 93, 95
burnout 150, 152

calm 97, 108
care experienced children 113, 149
cognitive behaviour therapy (CBT) 6, 10-11, 92, 104-107
cognitive restructuring 106, 112
combinatorial flexibility 78
common factors 103-104
common third, the 70
community participation 39
compassion fatigue 149-150, 152
connection 35, 165
COVID-19 4, 64
creativity: benefits of outdoors on 78-79; definition of 62; and depression 64; and early attachment 64; meeting psychological needs 65; unconditional positive regard and 139
critical incidents 128
critical reflection 127
Csikszentmihalyi, M. see flow
curiosity 54-55

DEARMAN 108-109
Deci and Ryan see self-determination theory
den building 122
depression 4-6; in children 53-54; CBT and depression 105; at work 150

dialectical behaviour therapy (DBT) 107-108, 114
discrimination 4, 162
dysregulation 8, 12, 108

early intervention 23
emotional labour 150, 152
emotional memories 33
emotional regulation 9, 26, 84, 91-92, 107, 135
empathy 40, 55, 110, 120
enculturation 40
environment-outdoor environment 77-78, 82; safe environment 54, 135

financial wellbeing 152
flow 65, 66, 73, 78, 86
forest school 79-80, 92
foucault 35
freud 6, 9
fun 43, 50, 85, 96

ghosts in the nursery 7
goleman *see* emotional memories
grief 8, 53

head, heart, hands 40, 42
hierarchy of needs 41, 44; *see* Maslow
hippocampus 23-24
hope 27-28

identity 4-5, 26, 38, 82, 109, 126, 139
income inequality 5-6
Iwama, Michael 127; *see also* Kawa River Model

journalling 136

key person 32, 37, 69-70
Kawa River Model 127

learning zone, the 50-51
life journeys 126-127
life story 126-127
life-world orientation 40, 56, 162
loneliness 4
loose parts 78

Maslow, A.H. 41, 44
mental health 12-13, 18, 147, 148; affecting young children 6-7; affects children's outcomes 153; effect of austerity on mental health 4, 5, 64, 65; impact of social media on 3, 6; increase in incidents of 3; increased awareness of 6; schools/education and mental health 4, 6, 143; mindfulness to support 91; outdoors positive effect on 82; parental 19, 33; play and mental health 49; PTSD and mental health 22; trauma and mental health 18; yoga and mental health 96; at work 148, 149, 157
mentalising 110-111
mindfulness 6, 90-99, 107-110
multiple affordances 78
music 62, 64, 65, 71, 73, 151, 162

Noddings, N. 38
non-verbal cues 133

PACE 54-56
persona dolls 10
person-centred 10; *see* Rogers, C.
Pestalozzi, J. H. 40, 44
physical health 5, 19, 49, 77, 148
PIESS 39
play: play and resilience 50, 52; risky play 50-51, 77-78; play therapy 52
prefrontal cortex 23
problem solving 26, 101
professional artistry 137
professional love 139, 152
progressive muscle relaxation 97
protective factors 26
psychodynamic approach 9-13

reflective writing 128
relationships: DBT to support 108; importance of 11, 26, 32, 44, 59, 69, 70, 74, 127, 135; impact of Aces on 19; impact of trauma on 22; listening 137; play and relationships 52, 54; outdoors and relationships 82, 110; stories for building relationships 120, 122; Theory of Mind and relationships 111; unconditional positive regard and relationships 140; work relationships 152, 153
relaxation 93, 95
resilience 19, 22, 25-27; and drama 67; outdoors 79; mindfulness 92; stories 119-121, 124; practitioner resilience 62, 71, 143, 153-154; *see also play and resilience*

Rogers, C. 10
Rogoff, B. 39, 44

safeguarding 11, 156
secondary traumatic stress 150
secure base 32, 35-36, 50
self-determination theory 42, 44, 65, 162
self-esteem 42
self-talk and affirmations 113, 157
shame 34, 43, 54
social capital 3, 5, 26
social deprivation 4
social media 6, 161
social pedagogy 50, 56, 65, 70, 152
stories 119-129
storytelling 128, 164
strange situation, the 32-33
strength based approaches 22
stress 83, 90-91, 94; vicarious trauma 149; recovery 84; stories to reduce 119; toxic 19-20, 23; In work environment 148, 150-153; in acceptance and commitment therapy 109; and yoga 96; Educational 4; and progressive muscle relaxation 97
supervision 54, 156

talking therapies 23, 102-104
theory of mind(tom) 110-111
toxic stress 19-20
toxic trio 19-20
trauma 22-25, 43, 71, 103; bibliotherapy and 120; effects on development 58; and identity 8; mindfulness to process 97, 103; need for specialist intervention 11, 54; use of PACE 55; and play 52; potential of creativity in recovery from 62-63, 68-69; and talking therapy 115; when nothing seems to help recovery from 70; and the outdoors 97; vicarious 149, 150
tree of life 127-128
trust/ trustful relationships 34, 36, 54, 135, 144, 148, 152

unconditional positive regard (UPG) 10, 133, 139, 164

Van der Kolk, Bessel 23
visualisation 94, 95, 115

withdrawal 34, 69, 104
workplace culture 148
worry management 105

yoga 23, 96

For Product Safety Concerns and Information please contact our EU representative GPSR@taylorandfrancis.com
Taylor & Francis Verlag GmbH, Kaufingerstraße 24, 80331 München, Germany

www.ingramcontent.com/pod-product-compliance
Lightning Source LLC
Chambersburg PA
CBHW080924300426
44115CB00018B/2938